The Female Body Bible

www.penguin.co.uk

The Female Body Bible

A Revolution in Women's Health and Fitness

Dr Emma Ross,
Baz Moffat and
Dr Bella Smith

The Well HQ

bantam

TRANSWORLD PUBLISHERS
Penguin Random House, One Embassy Gardens,
8 Viaduct Gardens, London SW11 7BW
www.penguin.co.uk

Transworld is part of the Penguin Random House group of companies whose addresses can be found at global.penguinrandomhouse.com

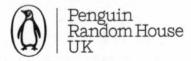

First published in Great Britain in 2023 by Bantam
an imprint of Transworld Publishers

A CIP catalogue record for this book
is available from the British Library.

ISBN 9781787636194

Text design by Couper Street Type Co.

Typeset in 12/16pt ITC Galliard Pro by Jouve (UK), Milton Keynes.
Printed and bound in Great Britain by Clays Ltd, Elcograf S.p.A.

The authorized representative in the EEA is Penguin Random House Ireland, Morrison Chambers, 32 Nassau Street, Dublin D02 YH68.

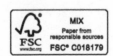

For those who want to forge a better
future for girls and women everywhere
– in sport, in health, in life.

Contents

Prologue

How We Became
The Well HQ

The Female Body Bible is the result of a collaboration between three women: Dr Emma Ross, Baz Moffat and Dr Bella Smith; a scientist, a fitness coach and a doctor – experts in our respective fields in women's health and fitness, and fervent practitioners who believe that body literacy is something every woman is entitled to.

Our mission is to ensure that everything that makes us extraordinarily female shouldn't be medicalized or considered niche, but be fully considered in making us fitter, healthier and happier humans. We want to make sure the conversation about women's experiences of their bodies, across their lives, goes mainstream. We want accessible, engaging information to reach all women, as well as everyone who supports, teaches, manages, trains or treats women. We want to overcome stigmas, reduce health inequities, address taboos and empower women to become architects of their own wellness, happiness and physicality.

Emma Ross is a PhD in exercise physiology who, after a decade as a science educator and researcher, became the Head of Physiology at the English Institute of Sport (EIS) and led the sports scientist team throughout the Rio and Tokyo Olympiads.

It was in this role that she launched the SmartHER project in 2016 to improve the support of female athletes within the high-performance sports system and was awarded the *Sunday Times* Sportswomen of the Year Changemaker award in 2021 for her work to improve sport for girls and women. Baz Moffat has a first class degree in sports science and a Masters in health-related behaviour change. She spent four years on the British Rowing team and after retiring, trained as a women's health coach, developing specialist expertise in pelvic health. Dr Bella Smith has been an NHS doctor for over twenty years, is a practice partner, and has qualified with specialisms in dermatology, women's health and menopause. She is an Ambassador for the Eve Appeal, the UK's Gynaecological Cancer Research Charity. Each of us has led a successful career in women's health for many years and is absolutely passionate about what she does. When mutual friends introduced us to each other, we soon realized our common goal – a desire to tackle the off-limits topics around women's health while educating and empowering women and those who support them. We all wanted to reimagine a future where no woman lacks knowledge and understanding of her body, across all her life stages, or lacks the confidence to use that knowledge to advocate for her own health and well-being. The Well HQ, as we call ourselves, is built on foundations of knowledge, credibility, science and experience, to support women on their journey from puberty to postmenopause.

This book, *The Female Body Bible*, is a distillation of what we've learned, giving you the tools you need to really understand your body, take control of your health and well-being, and harness your physiology and psychology to thrive in every aspect of your life. We've put our decades of experience of working with real women in the real world into these pages and we'd love to help you on your life journey, so read on to inform and empower yourself, and join in the conversation at www.thewell-hq.com.

Chapter 1

Mind the Gaps

'I will not take off my lipstick.'

It's 1967, and Kathrine Switzer is about to run the Boston Marathon by stealth. They don't allow women to run, because such a distance is thought to be too much for the fragile female body. Her coach is worried that she's put on earrings and lipstick, which will draw undue attention to the fact that she is female and get her dragged off the starting line. Kathrine Switzer doesn't remove her earrings, or her lipstick. But she does nearly get dragged from the marathon that day. At mile four, the race director Jock Semple tried to physically manhandle her out of the race. He failed, and Switzer went on to become the first woman to officially complete the Boston Marathon, which she did in four hours, twenty minutes.[1] In her account of that day, she recalls that as she ran, she wondered why more women had not tried to race before her.[2] She thought it was because they just didn't get the attraction of physical activity. But as she ran, she realized it wasn't that women didn't want to move, it was that they believed all the old myths, like that running ruined your reproductive organs or that it wasn't ladylike. She had a point: women had been discouraged from physical activity because medical professionals thought it dangerous, and the feminine ideal of the day didn't include such a sweaty and solitary habit as jogging. Our differences from men had been used to discourage us from moving our bodies. From that moment on, Switzer was determined to continue to break down the barriers to exercise for women.

But in the decades that followed, as women started to do more exercise and to compete, the differences that originally stopped them from taking part instead became overlooked and ignored completely.

The legacy of this oversight and the omission of understanding the female body has caused a significant issue in our health-conscious society: we have developed an enormous amount of information about training and exercise without taking into account the female-specific factors that are fundamental to every active woman getting the most out of her body and enjoying a dynamic, healthy life. Because for a long time, those features that make us biologically female have been regularly unspoken, ignored or dismissed. This information isn't being taught to girls in schools, it's not being taught to people who go on to work as health professionals, nor is it included in coaching or teaching qualifications.

While the identity of being sporty or active means different things to different people, our definition of being an active woman is someone who enjoys moving their body for health, fitness or performance reasons. It applies to someone who goes for regular walks, practises yoga at home, goes to gym classes, swims or works out at a health club, plays a team sport, is a CrossFitter or pursues ambitious endurance challenges. Anything that gets your heart rate up and makes you sweat a few times a week.

This disparity in knowledge when it comes to men's and women's health is what we're determined to change, through this book and in our work. We believe that everyone deserves to know more. That's why this isn't just a book, it's a movement – a call to action. Every woman deserves to know more about her body and everyone, regardless of their sex, needs to know more about women's bodies to remove the vestiges of secrecy and shame once and for all.

To kick off our journey through healthy, active womanhood we'd like you to join us in a pledge. It's a pledge that challenges the status quo for women. It's a commitment to refuse to accept systems that simply weren't designed for us to get the best out of ourselves.

Language

Vagina, periods, prolapse, menopause: as long as people wince at these words, women's issues will be discussed quietly in dark corners. But our bodies and their functions aren't embarrassing. There's a rich vocabulary around the female body, and it's high time it went mainstream.

Education

Women often don't know enough about their bodies and what to expect through various life stages. This leads to unease and a chronic lack of confidence. Greater understanding of your body and what you are likely to experience at certain points will help you identify issues and take appropriate action.

Perception

Health and fitness are not the same as aesthetics and being photogenic. Instead of prioritizing how a body looks, we need to focus on how it feels and functions. How it works. When we listen to the body, embrace it and nurture it, health and fitness will follow.

Women's welfare

We need a new rulebook – a cultural framework that supports, nurtures and empowers women. It needs to make knowledge about the female body – what's normal and what's not, what's appropriate and what's not, what's acceptable and what's non-negotiable – not just for women, but for everyone. We need to demand more of our employers, our institutions, our doctors, our coaches and trainers, our equipment and facilities, our gyms and our public toilets. OK is no longer OK. No more 'that's just the way it is'. We're tired of making do, it's time to make change.

Training

In sports science and medicine, as little as 6% of research is conducted exclusively on women.[3] Rewriting best practice for women will improve our health and fitness, and reduce the risk of injury. It will also improve our experiences of exercise and slash the dropout rate for women in sport. Big gains are achieved when women work out in tune with their bodies, rather than against them.

Not an exclusive club

This book is for any woman who moves her body; who aims to be fit and healthy throughout their life. Research shows that being active for 150 minutes per week at levels suitable to your age and fitness level is associated with reduced risk of suffering and dying from cardiovascular disease, cancer, respiratory diseases, neuro-degenerative diseases and metabolic conditions such as diabetes.[4] In women, higher fitness levels are associated with lower risk of death,[5] even among those with more body fat, meaning fitness is more important for health than fatness. If fitness were a pill, it would be a best-selling, market-leading sensation. Nothing else gets close to offering the lifelong health benefits of exercise.

It doesn't matter if you're dancing around the kitchen or running around the block, banging out the burpees at CrossFit or squeezing in some squats while burping the baby, moving is always a good idea. It's not about the label of 'athlete' or being a fitness fanatic; it's just about you knowing how to get enjoyment and satisfaction out of your active body. The knowledge we impart within these pages applies to every woman. The stories we've heard throughout our careers echo across all women.

The words we use

We want our work to support anyone who thinks they can benefit from learning about the female body, and how that connects to health, well-being and performance. Since talking about being female or being a woman can mean very different things to different people, we wanted to share what we mean when we use these terms in this book.

There is a difference between sex and gender. Someone's sex is biological – XX chromosomes make a female, and XY chromosomes make a male. Those genetics mean males and females are born with different anatomy and physiology. Gender is a combination of cultural, social, biological and psychological factors. It's how we look, act and feel. For many people, their biological sex aligns with their gender identity and this is often referred to as cisgender. In people whose biological sex and gender identity don't match, terminology varies, but it includes terms like transgender.

On the whole, our book relates to cisgender girls and women, and when we use the terms 'girls' and 'women' we are referring to people who were born with female genitals and who identify as women.

One of our missions is to shine a light on the fact that the research on, and understanding of, the female body is seriously lacking. Much of what we know about exercise, health and fitness is based on research conducted on males. This doesn't allow women to fulfil their potential, and we are dedicated to righting that wrong and empowering all active women with the knowledge and understanding to be architects of their own health and fitness.

Rising to the level of your goals

'We do not rise to the level of our goals. We fall to the level of our systems.'[6] You probably have goals for your fitness and health – perhaps it's to move more, drink less, or get better sleep. James Clear's book *Atomic Habits* suggests that goals are great for setting direction but designing a reliable system within your life is the best way to make successful progress.

A system is based on the habits you create in your life to help you live the way you want to. They can include not having caffeine after lunch, leaving your phone downstairs to make sure you sleep well, or putting your trainers and running kit by the side of the bed to ensure you get up for that early-morning jog. This book will help you create healthy habits that consider your whole body, where things like menstrual health, breast support, a female-centric approach to eating, pelvic health and life stages are all acknowledged and supported, so you can not only rise to, but exceed the level of your goals.

Mind the gaps

Before we design this new kick-ass system, we need to acknowledge that it's not quite as simple as just reading this book. There are a few fundamental gaps that mean even when we know what we need to know, we can't do what we need to do.

First there's the communication gap. We simply don't talk openly about many of the topics in this book. We don't tell our physiotherapist where we are in our menstrual cycle so they can see if our niggles are related to our hormones. We don't mention to our jogging group that we wet ourselves every week when everyone sprints back to the car park. We can often be found mumbling 'Why didn't anyone tell me?' as we bump into another inevitable yet unspoken aspect of womanhood. Increasingly, social media and campaigns like #metoo and #menopausematters drive an increased awareness of these issues, and a desire to discuss them. But undoubtedly, some stigma, embarrassment and discomfort remain, particularly between men and women, which is a dynamic that commonly exists across sport and physical activity. Whether it's a male Physical Education (PE) teacher, personal trainer or coach, only about 20% of women feel comfortable talking about female-specific issues with people in these roles;[7] and for the men, a lack of confidence in their knowledge is the biggest barrier to opening up the conversation.[8]

Then there's the data gap based on a lack of research on women in health, fitness, sport and exercise. When we started looking into this, years ago, a survey showed that as little as 4% of sports science research was conducted exclusively on women.[9] In 2020, when we felt like the world was wising up to the need for more research on women, we looked again. Over the intervening five years since the initial survey, we found that the dial had barely shifted, and that measly 4% had risen only to an embarrassing 6%.[10] That's worth repeating: only 6% of all sports science research in 2020 was conducted exclusively on women. And that's a problem, because most of the topics we cover in this book – the menstrual cycle, breast support, high prevalence of stress incontinence, menopause – relate exclusively to the female body.

Outside of that tiny percentage of female-only research, 60%

is done on mixed-participant groups of both males and females. This work fails to serve anyone well but is most challenging for women because the changing physiology and psychology across the menstrual cycle is usually ignored. It's so important for women to get curious about the research that underpins what we believe to be true, and which informs any actions we take based on 'the science'. Often, the findings from research simply don't apply to us, or only apply to us for a few days of our monthly cycle. To give you an idea of how important that can be: long after they were released for safe use in all patients, new research showed that the effectiveness and, in some cases, the safety of antihistamines, antipsychotics, antibiotics and heart medication was affected by the menstrual cycle.[11]

The gender data gap can often be hidden in plain sight. When research is conducted exclusively on males, it's not made clear that this research applies only to men; instead, the implication is that the findings will be relevant for everyone. At a recent conference for PE teachers and coaches of school sport, Emma sat through a presentation on the importance of effectively recognizing and treating concussion in school sport – a hot topic. Yet all the data presented was from boys' sport. Worryingly, there is emerging evidence that girls report concussion more frequently, and with worse symptoms than boys. But in this case, the guidance for all sports teachers was based on findings derived entirely from male subjects, without acknowledging this. We must demand that research transparently states who it was performed on and to whom its findings best apply, and we must ensure that guidance in sport and exercise that applies to girls and women is based on research performed on girls and women.

Without wishing to sound ungrateful, it's also important to note that the 6% of research that is performed exclusively on girls and women is not all that good. In a comprehensive analysis of all research conducted on the menstrual cycle and performance in sport and exercise, when the studies were rated against rigorous criteria, only 8% of them were found to be of high enough quality for the outcomes to be trusted.[12] A survey of ten years' worth of research on strength training in women found that only three studies[13] used research methods that met the highest industry standard.

But it's not all bad news. There are some brilliant people working on high-quality research in women's sport, health and fitness in the UK and around the world, and their work has been used to inform the pages of this book.

A key step to drive change should be to take research from the pages of hallowed academic journals and translate it quickly into what we do on the gym floor, what we put on our dinner plate, and organizations' HR policies. But it's the translation of this research into practice that often forms the bottleneck: it's thought that in healthcare, it takes about seventeen years.[14] This is the final, often most impactful gap: the 'doing' gap.

It's one thing to know all the stuff in this book, and quite another to put it into practice, or to share the knowledge with the girls and women in your life. How many of us know that screen time before bed is the devil when it comes to sleeping well, but still find ourselves having a quick scroll of the socials before lights out? How many of us know that we should do our pelvic floor exercises every day, but don't because we're not actually sure what to do and why it's so vital. Even in the upper echelons of sport, athletes and trainers know there are some important female-specific things they should be considering but they aren't really sure what to do about them. In a study of the top five US colleges, only 3% of sports coaches who were working with women said they felt like they actually trained their athletes in a female-centric way that honoured the important differences from the male athletes they coached. They didn't know how to turn what they had learned into tangible actions in their everyday approach to sport and exercise.[15] Our ambition for this book is that it makes you feel empowered and equipped to take action.

Who are *we* to say?

If there isn't enough reliable research currently available, how can we write a credible, evidence-based book to help you learn what you need to know to be well? There are definitely times when the lack of evidence means we don't know enough to have developed a gold-standard approach. For example, there's some exciting research that shows the benefits of doing different exercises in sync with your menstrual cycle, but it's not a large enough body of evidence to become mainstream advice. There's also some interesting research into the links between injuries and our hormones, but some of it simply isn't of good enough quality to make use of yet.

That said, we have drawn from the best research available, established wisdom and our own practice-based evidence following decades of experience as a scientist, a doctor and a coach each working with thousands of women. This is not intended to be the big book of rules for being an active woman. For each of the topics we cover in this book, there isn't a one-size-fits-all approach that will be true for everyone. All women will experience their body in the context of their life, their age, their relationships, their health, their work, sport and leisure pursuits. We are each a unique combination of our nature and nurture. Don't ever be hoodwinked into believing that what works perfectly for one woman will work wonders for you too.

While this isn't the rulebook, it *is* the playbook. It's a book of all the elements that go into getting the most out of your body, and a selection of strategies that you can try to find out what works for you and your incredible body.

Chapter 2

Health and Fitness Through a Female Filter

The 'shrink it and pink it' model seems to have been applied to women's health and fitness; it's assumed that what works for the male body will probably work just fine for the female body too. Women are offered pink versions of men's kit, are served up the same type of training – albeit with lighter weights and lower targets – and are told to approach nutrition in the same way as men, but just eat less. Well, you know what they say about the word 'assume'? It makes an 'ass' out of 'u' and 'me', and that's certainly true here. Now that we know better, we have an opportunity to do better when it comes to our approach to being active women.

Instead of adapting what already exists in a system of sport and exercise that has been designed by men, for men, we'd like the entire approach to be reinvented with training programmes, kit, classes and facilities specifically designed to meet women's needs. We'd like a female filter applied to the landscape of sport and exercise. This chapter introduces some of the important factors we think need to be considered in our new world order. These are the things we want to be better understood by women who are exercising, training or competing.

The menstrual cycle

Without a doubt, this should be considered one of the most important areas for a girl or woman to understand because, for the vast majority of women in the world, the menstrual cycle is a defining rhythm of their life.

The ebb and flow of menstrual cycle hormones affects us physically and emotionally. These hormones are amazing for our short- and long-term health, and they have an impact on how we feel about moving our bodies too, yet we don't instinctively know how to have the best experience of our cycle, and what we're taught at school as young adults is not enough. We need more than biology, because a theoretical description is meaningless unless it connects with what women actually experience. If we're encouraged to notice how we're feeling, how there is a rhythm to our cycle that we can work with to minimize the effect of symptoms and to optimize the times when we feel terrific, that adds a whole new dimension to our life. It means that we're not pushing the cart uphill, by eating, exercising and resting in a way that tunes in to our physiology and how we experience it. It also means that if we do have to perform on days where our cycle symptoms show up, then we have strategies in place to overcome them, and still get the best out of ourselves.

The menstrual cycle is a superpower – but all too often it is not described as such, which is at best a shame and at worst a drastic oversight of the potential girls and women gain through understanding their cycle.

Hormonal contraception

Not all women will experience a natural menstrual cycle all the time, because about 50% of women will use hormonal contraception – most commonly the pill – at some stage.[1] As with all medications, it's sensible to make sure that you're making an informed decision about what's right for you, and what to do if you don't find the right fit the first time. Yet hormonal contraception is not something we're well educated about; instead, we tend to resort to friends' reports of what's worked for them or we simply use the first thing we're prescribed. What's more, hormonal contraceptives still come with a 'try it and see' approach, which can make finding the one that's right for you hard work.

Hormonal contraceptives are popular because they are effective and convenient. They are also a great solution for many women suffering with debilitating menstrual cycle issues or underlying conditions. However, we think that we should all be better informed about all forms of hormonal contraception, their side effects, what might best suit our body and how they might impact our lives.

Simply knowing the ins and outs of using the pill can make us better ambassadors for our health. For example, in sport, having a period as part of a natural menstrual cycle is a sign that a woman is getting enough energy through her diet to fuel her training. Hormonal contraceptive users don't get that monthly high five from their period, as the withdrawal bleeds on the pill – bleeding in response to days when the pill doesn't include hormones – are not the same as the bleeding experienced during a period. Yet we've met lots of active women who didn't know that using hormonal contraceptives can mask a sport-related cycle dysfunction, such as under-fuelling or over-training.

For active women, the side effects of using hormonal contraceptives might be challenging, from weight gain and low mood to reductions in performance. It's time we had more open conversations and education about hormonal contraception in the context of our active lives and our sporting goals.

Breast support

The first patent for a sports bra was granted in 1979, but we've still got a long way to go in terms of this essential piece of kit. Breast support has been hugely overlooked – thrown into the underwear category, rather than considered to be a functional, performance-impacting bit of kit. Ask any active woman how essential a good bra is and she'll tell you in a heartbeat.

Thankfully the evidence backs this up and shows the significant performance gains that can be had purely by properly supporting a woman's breasts. Whether it's about alleviating pain and discomfort, making exercise feel easier or reducing the energy cost of your movement, the right breast support is proven to make a difference.[2]

The challenge at the moment is that although innovation and technology exists, and brands are making brilliant sports bras, these are not getting into the hands (or should we say on to the breasts) of all women. Whether that's because of their often extortionate price tag or the lack of understanding about which design and fit of bra would be suitable for your body and your sport, there are still lots of women without the right breast support.

Poor breast support is holding girls and women back. From the 46% of teens who have concerns about their breasts and exercise that stop them participating in sport[3] to the fact that women with a D-cup or larger breast size do 37% less exercise because of their breasts[4] there are multiple reasons we need to be teaching all girls and women how to choose a sports bra that fits properly, regardless of their breast size and budget. We would love to see all sports stores having trained sports bra fitters so that, just as you would hop on an in-store treadmill to see if a pair of trainers is right for you, you could get sound advice before buying the sports bra that's right for you.

Pelvic floor

We all have a pelvic floor and for many of us it comes into sharp focus around childbirth, but the stats from sport and exercise will blow your mind. Most women who participate in high-impact sports, such as netball, gymnastics and running, leak during training or competition because their pelvic floors are not working as they should do. This might just be the last taboo in women's health, especially for those keen on exercise, because if you can train every day, perform at a high level or run fast, why can't your body do something really basic like stay continent?

Mums and midlife women have 'permission' to have pelvic floor issues, but young athletic women often feel they do not, which means that they rarely reach out to get help. The reason young women have pelvic floor dysfunction is usually different from post-natal or menopausal women, but a basic understanding of how to activate, relax and coordinate the pelvic floor muscles can help women of all ages maintain or restore good pelvic floor health.

It's key that pelvic floor dysfunction is not quietly accepted in the context of sport and exercise – it's not OK to laugh off sneezy wees, leaky bouncing, the number of trips to the toilet you've taken or the fact that you have to wear black to hide the leaks. We need to move towards a place where everyone can have open conversations about this topic, know how training can be adapted to help restore good pelvic floor function and know where to find the local women's health physiotherapist to get additional support.

Injury risk

Women are up to six times more likely to suffer a non-contact anterior cruciate ligament (ACL) injury in the knee than men[5] and twice as likely in other joints in our body.[6] Despite the reasons for injury being complex and varied, what is clear is that we need to design training programmes so that girls and women don't get injured as often.

There is growing evidence to support a gendered approach to warming up: if girls and women do ten minutes of specific conditioning exercises three times a week, then injury risk is reduced by over 40%.[7] Examples of these exercises can be found in the FIFA '11+' football warm-up, or the England Netball 'Jump High Land Strong' programme, both of which can be used by anyone of any age and not just footballers or netballers. There are also some great resources if you search 'ACL injury prevention for females' on YouTube (look for videos developed by sports scientists, physiotherapists and orthopaedic and sports medicine clinics). These programmes promote injury resilience by using conditioning exercises to address some of the key risk factors that have been found in women – muscle weakness, muscle imbalance, poor landing mechanics and lack of agility or instinctive awareness of where parts of our body are without looking at them, known as proprioception. All of these factors can be modified through proper training to stop them contributing to injury risk. We've met so many women whose participation in a sport they love has been cut short because of a significant injury. Let's change the course of future generations of women by helping them develop strong, resilient bodies that move well.

Strength training

Over the course of our lives as women, staying strong and resilient means we can stay active, healthy and happy. Strength training is a really important component of a balanced approach to fitness, especially for women as they enter midlife, when muscle strength and bone density can be compromised by declining hormones. If you've never done weights, you don't have to head to the gym; home-based workouts will work well. Whether you do exercises like squats, arm curls and shoulder presses, either with a two-litre milk carton or with dumbbells, barbells or kettlebells, the key is that it should be a challenge – it should feel like work; this way your body will adapt and get stronger. So many women feel intimidated by strength training that they never pursue it. We need the culture around strength training to shift, and for it to welcome and educate girls and women of all ages.

Nutrition

Most women get nutrition wrong – we know this sounds negative, but it's true. It's for a whole host of reasons, including the fact that most nutritional advice, even when it's 'evidence'-based, is taken from research done on men. A great example is intermittent fasting or fasted training, which works well for a male's physiology but is not effective in females, and actually has a potentially harmful impact on our physiology. Then there's the fact that improving gut health can be more impactful for women, based on emerging research showing that it's more tightly linked to immune function and hormone health in women than it is in men.

If the female filter were applied in our brave new world, we'd ensure that everyone knew that:

- without a balanced approach to nutrition, it doesn't matter how much you train, study or work, you won't be able to achieve your full potential
- eating the right food allows us to adapt to the stimulus of exercise; without getting enough energy from our diet, we compromise our performance and our health; we see so many cases of athletes who end up breaking, either

physically or emotionally, simply because they haven't been getting their nutrition right

- educating girls about the importance of a balanced diet will help them become strong, resilient women who have a healthy relationship with food, exercise and their bodies
- nutrition helps us manage the symptoms our body throws at us; there are inherent qualities in certain foods that help women's health challenges; eating a diet rich in anti-inflammatory[8] foods such as seeds, berries, turmeric, garlic and ginger, and having foods rich in micronutrients such as calcium, magnesium, zinc, B and D vitamins, have been shown to alleviate menstrual and perimenopausal symptoms[9]

To achieve this, we need reliable sources of information that don't prey on a woman's insecurities around her shape, weight or size and which delve deeper into her health and well-being on a level that is concerned about how she functions, rather than how she looks.

Mindset

Let's start with a disclaimer: there's no such thing as a male brain or a female brain. Our brains are all beautifully unique and are sculpted by our genetics and our biology – that's the nature bit – and by our education, our families, our cultures and our experiences – that's the nurture bit. But most women will say that they often think or behave in different ways to men, and most men will say the same. Research confirms this, and it gives us clues to how we can use our mindset to get the best out of ourselves and others in sport and exercise.

One interesting difference is how women derive confidence and motivation to pursue their goals. Women tend to draw on the quality of their relationships with the people that support them – their teacher, trainer or teammates. Men are usually driven more by the quality of the achievements of the people who support them, and how successful they've been helping others achieve their goals. If this resonates with you, it's more likely that in the pursuit of your goals, you'll benefit from being supported by someone who cares about you as a person rather than someone who is a technically brilliant master.

We also know that women are more motivated by personal development, by mastery and by each other, compared with men, who tend to have a more egocentric approach – they are motivated by winning and by beating others. Considering this might help us find an approach to health, fitness and performance that keeps us coming back and putting in the effort because it's pressing all the right buttons in the brain.

Training across the lifespan

It's impossible to design our new world of health and physical activity without considering the life stages a woman goes through, from the inevitable changes of puberty and menopause – which impact us physiologically, psychologically and socially – to those brought about through pregnancy and birth. Whether you have experienced all of them or just some, each reader will have had a very different lived experience of each one.

These life stages are often vulnerable moments in a woman's life in terms of her relationship with sport and exercise; they are times when her body changes hugely. The experience can be traumatic. They can also be times when women do not feel in control of what's happening to them, physically or emotionally. Current research shows that many girls and women stop exercising or fall out of love with sport at these points in their lives. Our female-centric Utopia would provide for women's physical and emotional health at each of these stages by better educating women of all ages about the long-term benefits of staying active throughout their lives and by creating systems that make being active an accessible and enjoyable way to live.

Changing the world

It doesn't matter how much we learn about our bodies and how to optimize our exercise routines, if the world doesn't change, we will all be limited by the male-centric system. A system that doesn't acknowledge and support female bodies, that continues to generate data and evidence based on men, that continues to stigmatize topics like periods and pelvic floors, that values being photogenic over health and happiness. And while changing the world may sound like a grand plan, if we all play a part, we can make it happen.

When it comes to sport and fitness at school, at work or in the gym, we need to create psychologically safe environments. These don't just benefit women, they benefit everyone. Psychological safety means being able to speak up about whatever is going on with you and what is getting in the way of you participating or performing that day, and not being afraid that you will be judged, dismissed, or that speaking up will have negative consequences. A psychologically safe environment is one where girls and women believe that those around them will be comfortable talking about all the topics we cover in this book. It's a compassionate environment where we listen, validate, empathize and commit to support. And before anyone pursuing ambitious goals assumes that this type of environment could become too comfortable, psychological safety can still exist with accountability, ambition and high performance. These are not mutually exclusive ideals.

It's an *Avengers Assemble* kind of situation, one where researchers, educational institutions, sports coaches, trainers, teachers, parents, brands, governing bodies, and of course girls and women, can all play a role in forging a future where girls and women feel that they truly belong; that any place they decide to spend their time has been designed with them in mind. That they have been provided with enough education about their bodies, throughout their lives, for their body, and how they experience it, not to be the thing that holds them back from fulfilling their potential in work, sport – and life.

Chapter 3

Mastering Your Menstrual Cycle

The menstrual cycle is incredible. It's the defining biological rhythm of half our lives as women. Yet information about the cycle is often distilled into reproductive biology lessons, where we learn about fallopian tubes and maturing eggs, about ovulation and uterus linings, rather than its power and influence over us throughout our lives. Our personal relationship with our cycle is often focused on how awful it makes us feel at certain times of the month, or how annoying it is when your period arrives on the first day of your long-awaited beach holiday. Yet there is so much more to the cycle that we want everyone to know.

We believe that knowing more about the menstrual cycle:

- is fundamental to lifelong health and well-being in women
- gives us important, reassuring and empowering context to our lives
- gives us an opportunity to stop our bodies holding us back
- can help young women navigate puberty when the influence of newly cycling hormones can feel confusing and chaotic
- can better prepare women for starting a family and help improve awareness of how our bodies cope in the aftermath of birth

- can prepare and empower women through their peri- and post-menopausal years
- can be an important part of our approach to fitness and getting the best out of our body throughout all stages of life
- can change your life

Yet the general level of understanding of our cycle is notoriously low. In 2019 the Royal College of Obstetricians and Gynaecologists reported that women are 'woefully uneducated at every life stage' about what's happening in their bodies and how that relates to their physical and mental health and well-being.[1] In a study of 14,000 active women, 72% said they had never had any education about exercise and their menstrual cycle.[2]

Emma

After barely hearing the word 'period' for the whole decade I worked in Olympic and Paralympic sport, I am on a mission to take the menstrual cycle mainstream and one of my first jobs is to stop people using euphemisms. There are over 5,000 words used to mean 'period' across the globe. The volume alone is enough to tell us that we don't like talking openly about menstruation. When it comes to our sexual anatomy and our reproductive functions, we have for centuries tried to find other words to describe them. We're happy to talk about breathing and sweating, nipples and belly buttons, but when it comes to vulvas, vaginas and periods, there are so many euphemisms that it's easy to lose track of whether someone is talking about their vulva or their pet pony, their period or the title of a horror film. Social anthropologists explain that euphemisms don't typically exist for bodily functions without histories of stigma. They persist because there hasn't been a good enough reason to correct them: why get rid of words which make us feel less uncomfortable about things that we believe are vulgar or embarrassing? When we describe breathing or sweating, the words don't create emotional tension, embarrassment or disgust. Professor Chris Bobel, a researcher in the field of sociology of menstruation, goes further, suggesting that as well as exposing our social views, euphemisms also reflect how distant we are from our bodies. When we teach children euphemisms, we start a lifetime of skirting around the realities of our body, and body literacy is hard to come by when you don't even have the right language to describe it.[3]

Yes, I'm hormonal. So try to keep up!

The term 'hormonal' has been exclusively reserved for women, particularly in the days before their period. The word has been entangled with our emotionality, which is often seen as a weakness. Being 'hormonal' is considered an apology. When you react emotionally to something, perhaps by snapping at someone, or if you feel low, you may say, 'Sorry, I'm a bit hormonal today.' Please stop apologizing for your hormones. Hormones are amazing, and none of us would be alive without them.

When we dismiss women's emotions in the days before their period (well, any time, actually) as hormonal, we are effectively deeming them invalid. Yes, hormones can affect our mood, and yes, they can make the highs higher and the lows lower, but (in the absence of mental health issues) these feelings are caused by something real and valid, and you shouldn't deny them.

In sport we're accustomed to tuning in to and taking advantage of the effects of hormones. Take the practice of 'priming' by male athletes.[4] In the hour leading up to a football or rugby match, the coach makes a rousing speech to his players, they watch footage of them beating the team they're about to play, they beat their chests, or do some push-ups on the changing-room floor. These activities cause a natural spike in testosterone, so that these players can capitalize on the effects of this hormone – it helps make them aggressive, strong, self-confident and more inclined to take risks during the game. But, if these feelings spill over and we see a player commit a foul, a late tackle, or talk back to the referee in the first few minutes of the game, we don't hear the commentator say, 'Oooh, he's hormonal,' do we? Yet if we were to describe that player's response, in physiological terms, it would be a hormonal response. The fact is that all humans are hormonal, all the time. Hormones keep our bodies working properly, responding to what we're doing and what the world around us is doing.

When it comes to our menstrual cycle, our two main cycle hormones – oestrogen and progesterone – exert their influence throughout our body, from muscles to gut, bones to brain. These hormones not only control our cycle and our ability to reproduce, they have widespread effects on everything from our growth and development, to our metabolism, mood, immune function, body temperature, sleep and cognitive functions. When we think about how hormone levels rise and fall across a cycle, impacting on the body and the brain, it comes as no surprise that women often feel different when levels are high compared with when they are low.

Four steps to menstrual cycle domination

When it comes to the menstrual cycle, there are whole books written on the subject. In this chapter, we've distilled our approach to understanding the menstrual cycle into four steps:

- knowing what the menstrual cycle is, what's considered healthy and normal, and how best to manage it
- understanding and tracking your own unique experience of the cycle
- managing your symptoms
- training around your cycle for improved fitness or performance

There is no right or wrong way for you to explore your cycle, and you might only want to take the first two or three steps. It's your cycle, and the fact that you are seeking to understand more means you are already improving your body literacy, and that's a personal revolution in itself.

Step 1: Know what's normal

As the L'Oréal ad says, here comes the science bit. The menstrual cycle is a predictable pattern of hormonal fluctuation across roughly twenty-eight days. While we know for certain what the cycle looks like as a hormonal pattern, there is actually a lot of variation between women in terms of the levels of hormones we each produce, our ability to metabolize these hormones and our sensitivity to them. Factors such as lifestyle, sleep, diet, type and amount of physical activity, as well as illness and injury, can also influence the release and effect of the cycle hormones in our bodies. This means that no two women's cycle experiences are likely to be the same. However, with that in mind, like all the topics we cover in this book, a great place to start is to know what's normal and what's not.

The menstrual cycle 101

- Having a regular, manageable period is a vital sign of whole-body health in menstruating women.[5]
- Girls should start their periods by the age of sixteen. The average age for starting (in the UK) is twelve.
- The first day of your period is day one of your menstrual cycle.
- Periods usually last between five to seven days.
- During a healthy period we can lose anywhere between 30ml and 50ml of blood.
- A regular tampon can hold about 5ml of blood.
- You are considered to have heavy periods if you lose over 80ml of menstrual blood during your period.
- Some women have very regular cycles that are exactly the same length each month, but for some women their cycle length can vary by up to eight days per month, and that's normal too.
- Two important hormones are released by your ovaries during your cycle: oestrogen and progesterone. They peak and trough across your cycle and send signals across your body.
- The first half of your cycle is called the follicular phase and includes your period, with oestrogen rising from day one of your period until ovulation.
- The second half of your cycle is called the luteal phase, when progesterone and oestrogen are both elevated before rapidly declining just before your next period arrives.
- Ovulation, which is the release of an egg from the ovary, happens about midway through your cycle. Your hormones help your body to know when to release the egg.

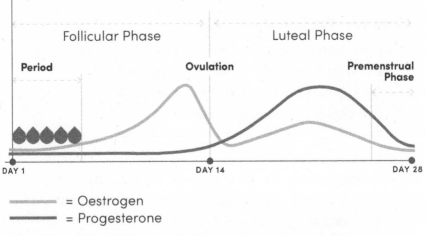

The menstrual cycle, showing fluctuations of oestrogen and progesterone

The cycle starts in the brain

Although we usually focus on the two hormonal stars of the menstrual cycle – oestrogen and progesterone, which are mainly produced in the ovaries – there are other hormones that influence whether a woman has a healthy cycle that originate far away from the female reproductive system, in the hypothalamus gland in the brain.

A healthy cycle includes a period and ovulation. At the start of a cycle, the hypothalamus sends a message to the pituitary gland, telling it to release important signalling hormones called follicle stimulating hormone and luteinizing hormone. These help the body choose a dominant follicle from our ovaries, which will be 'the chosen one' to release its egg during this cycle, usually around twelve to fourteen days after the first day of the period. Just prior to ovulation, there is a surge in luteinizing hormone that causes this chosen egg to burst out of its follicle and be released from the ovary. This is called ovulation, and the follicle that once held the egg now turns into a temporary gland for the rest of the cycle, called the corpus luteum, which releases oestrogen and progesterone across the second half of the cycle. Isn't that amazing? The follicle that houses the egg takes on another job, as a hormone-producing gland, after its first job of egg storage is made redundant.

This brain-to-ovary signalling network is very important and can be impacted by what we eat, how much we exercise and how we manage stress. When our brain senses that all is not well in our body, the signals it sends to our ovaries to keep the menstrual cycle running smoothly can be disturbed, which can have all sorts of knock-on effects.

The big 'O'

Ovulation is a vital part of a healthy cycle, but it's hard to know whether it's happening or not, because unlike the period, there's nothing to see during ovulation. However, up to 40% of women know they're ovulating because they experience ovulation pain.[6] This can alternate each month from the left to the right side, depending on which ovary is ovulating; but though it was once assumed that ovaries took turns in releasing the month's egg, this isn't necessarily the case. Another way women know they are ovulating is by noticing changes in their cervical fluid (vaginal discharge). If your cervical fluid is clear and stretchy like egg white (as opposed to dry and sticky, or very watery), it indicates you are around ovulation time. Your body cleverly produces this type of cervical fluid around ovulation as it helps to keep sperm healthy and assists them on their journey to the newly released egg.

Ovulation triggers production of the other important cycle hormone, progesterone. The arrival of this hormone helps prepare your uterus for the implantation of a fertilized egg. Those not wishing to get pregnant may be pleased to know progesterone also regulates blood pressure and improves mood and sleep. Without ovulation and the production of progesterone, our cycle becomes unbalanced and unhealthy.

So, why wouldn't we ovulate, if the point of the cycle is to release an egg so that we can get pregnant? When our body is under extreme stress, whether physical or emotional, it starts to shut down those functions that aren't essential to keep us alive – and reproductive capability is one of the first things to go. An example we see all too often is in active girls and women who expend a lot of energy doing a high volume of exercise and not regularly replacing that energy with good nutrition. When this happens, the reproductive cycle may begin to shut down. At first ovulation stops, but the period remains; eventually, though, under continued imbalance between energy expenditure and food intake, periods disappear too, and the cycle is completely suppressed, which is very unhealthy.

Unwanted symptoms of the cycle might be a sign that the important act of ovulation hasn't gone according to plan. For example, heavy periods can be caused by too much oestrogen, which builds up the lining of the uterus,[7] and not enough progesterone, whose job is to stop that build-up.

There will be blood

The first day of a woman's cycle is marked by the start of menstrual bleeding. In a healthy cycle, bleeding shouldn't be so heavy that you have to change a traditional period product, like a tampon or pad, more than every three or four hours. If you are soaking through products more quickly, it's likely that you suffer from heavy periods. Period management is often overlooked. Tampons and pads are dished out to pubescent girls with some vague instructions for use, yet as health and sports practitioners we talk to teenagers all the time who struggle to use tampons and don't want to ask for help. When we deliver workshops in schools, real questions from fourteen-year-old girls include 'How do I know if I've put my tampon in the right hole?', 'How do I put my tampon in so it stays there?' and 'Can I wear a period pad in the swimming pool?' You know how there's a 'Resuscitation Annie' dummy who helps millions of people learn vital first aid?

Well, what about a 'Period Patty' equivalent, to help girls learn about their anatomy and how to insert tampons?

Finding the right period product to suit the activity you are doing, the kit you have to wear and what's most comfortable to perform in – possibly for hours at a time – depends on many factors, yet we often just use products that our mothers told us about years ago. But there are so many different products on the market these days that it's worth checking out what's now available. These include:

- conventional tampons and pads, which have had an environmental and component make-over, giving women the option to buy products that are better for their bodies and the planet
- reusable tampon applicators that can last a lifetime and save thousands of plastic applicators ending up in the oceans[8]
- menstrual cups, which are inserted vaginally and collect, rather than absorb, your period. They are often plastic-free, made from materials like silicone, and can be reused month after month
- the new kid on the block: period underwear – underpants with a built-in super-thin absorbent lining (just 3mm thick) that can hold up to three or four tampons' worth of blood
- or the same thing but better still: period underwear that can be worn for twenty-four hours leak-free, since the built-in absorbent gusset can hold up to ten tampons' worth of blood

Bloody marvellous. Period underwear in particular is the revolution that women have been waiting for. These products are also now designed for active women, with movement and sweat in mind (think wicking fabrics), and period-pant brands are partnering with sports brands. These are such a great solution for all girls and women who do sport and exercise, but particularly when you are out of range of a toilet, such as going on a long bike ride, running a marathon, playing cricket or sailing. The initial up-front cost can feel high when compared with your average box of tampons, but when you weigh up how much you'll save over the course of your menstruating years, it's a great swap to make, both financially and environmentally.

One of our favourite things to show women, particularly teenage girls, is period swimwear. 'How does it work?' they cry. We don't know. As far as we're concerned, it really is magic, sent from a female entrepreneur who needed the world to up its period product game. There aren't many on the market at the time of writing,[9] but we hope that now some brands are leading the way, others will soon follow. Because period swimwear is a game changer. There are so many girls and women who don't want to use tampons or can't get to grips with them, and for them swimming is simply off the table when they're on their period. Not any more!

Another helpful innovation is a bag to keep your used products safely sealed away, which you can pop in a handbag or pocket without fear of anything smelling or leaking.[10] Because there isn't always a bin, is there? Women who like camping or hiking, or who compete in sports where portable toilets are the norm, as well as girls doing Duke of Edinburgh expeditions, all find this invention useful when trying to manage periods. Such bags also stop the 'flushers' among us and create more 'binners'. That's important because many tampons come wrapped in plastic, are encased in plastic applicators, and have plastic strings dangling from one end, while many even include a thin layer of plastic in the absorbent part – yet more than half of tampon users still flush their used products and applicators. Flushing our period products means that the many plastics they contain block our sewers and pollute our rivers, oceans and beaches – a recent report cited an average of 4.8 pieces of menstrual waste per 100m of beach cleaned in the UK.[11]

Step 2: Understand the experience of your own cycle

Each woman's menstrual cycle is beautifully unique. Now you know what's within the range of normality for a healthy cycle, you can start to really explore your personal experience.

When we think about how our cycle hormones affect us, it's useful to remember that this is a reproductive cycle. Hormones don't just help women become pregnant and nurture a new embryo, they also help women behave in a way that is most likely to find a mate, have sex at the right time, and then back off and relax as the baby grows.

Of course, many women don't wish to get pregnant each month, but that doesn't mean our hormones aren't still influencing us to that end. The good news is that these are transferable behaviours – if you're not actively trying to get pregnant, your hormones can still be harnessed to help your work productivity and exercise habits.

Tracking your cycle

No one can tell you what your cycle experience will be. That's unique to you. Yet women don't always know where they actually are in their cycle, and they often can't tell you with absolute clarity which of their physical or emotional symptoms are linked to their cycle. Tracking your cycle, noting when your period starts and finishes and any symptoms you may experience, is the key to understanding its impact on you and doing so can catalyse many possibilities for experiencing your training, work and other aspects of your life in new ways. By learning to read your body, the way it feels when things are right or wrong, what's normal for you and whether that's actually normal at all, you can begin to make the most of your cycle.

One of the most important things that cycle tracking allows you to do is to anticipate what your cycle is going to throw at you – good and bad. Once you've tracked for a few months, you will have greater insight into how you feel physically and emotionally at different points of your cycle, and, by a process of elimination, be able to establish what's not related to your cycle at all. Anticipating what's coming puts you in the driving seat, rather than having your cycle control you. That's a total power shift, and for many women that's very empowering in itself.

Knowing what's coming is acknowledged to be a key factor in building resilience. Resilience is the ability to respond to what is happening by changing how you approach it or doing something differently. Developing menstrual cycle resilience is one of the greatest things you can do as a woman. It's knowing what you need and when you need it to get the best experience of your cycle, so that you get the most out of your life.

Emma

After I had my first child, I started suffering strange recurring bouts of nausea, diarrhoea and overwhelming fatigue. My doctor was stumped by what could be causing these symptoms and eventually referred me to a tropical disease clinic. The first question the consultant asked me was where I had been to pick up a suspected tropical disease. Um . . . nowhere. I had a baby nine months ago – I've barely been dressed, let alone been anywhere tropical! I was sent away from the clinic, unsurprisingly none the wiser. After the symptoms kept flaring up, I saw another doctor, the first female doctor I had seen. I don't know whether that played a role in her ability to diagnose me, but she quickly linked my symptoms and the regularity with which they were appearing with potential cycle-related issues. I started tracking my cycle, and it immediately became clear she was right. It turned out I had severe premenstrual symptoms that would flare up the day before my period arrived. And the good news was there were things that could be done to help. (In my case, first non-steroidal anti-inflammatories, which helped a bit, followed by the progesterone-only pill for a couple of years, which took away the symptoms completely. Better still, when I came off it, I didn't get the symptoms at all any more.) What enraged me most about this experience was that a previous doctor had considered a rare tropical illness before considering premenstrual syndrome (PMS), and for so long my symptoms weren't even validated; rather, they were dismissed as being in my head, or completely normal.

When it comes to our menstrual cycle, it's really easy to miss what can turn out to be fairly obvious connections. But there's little chance your doctor will link anything to your cycle unless you go with your tracking notes in hand.[12] Tracking your cycle not only makes you the architect of your cycle experience, but also the best ambassador for your cycle health.

Tracking can seem like yet another thing to do, or something you might forget to do and then beat yourself up about. You might doubt it will even tell you anything anyway. That's why it's so important that you find a method that suits you. Cycle tracking is a deliberate action to invest in your menstrual, physical and emotional health, and it does take some time and effort. But if you approach it with the right mindset – hopeful and curious about what it will reveal to you, and excited by how it can empower you – then you will be pleasantly surprised by the results.

Keep it simple
The mechanism of tracking the cycle doesn't need to be complicated. The main thing is that you must understand and value

why you are doing it, otherwise it's unlikely to be a habit that sticks. When you first start tracking, you'll forget on some days, or you might only remember to mark down your period, or only your symptoms in the days before your period. That's OK, it gets easier the longer you do it, and the more tracking tells you about your cycle, the more motivated you'll be to log consistently and regularly. Even just tracking when your period arrives each time will start to give you an idea of your cycle length and how regular that is from month to month.

Remember that cycle regularity is a good indicator of lifelong health. You can reflect on what and whether anything has had an influence on your cycle's regularity. Collect information that's important to you and keep it simple. You could just use one word each day, make notes in a calendar or rate symptoms out of five. Whatever you do, give yourself permission to take a breath, pause for twenty seconds and check in with yourself, your body and how you feel each day. Once you start tracking, it's surprising how, instead of brushing off how you feel, you'll want to note something down to see if it's related to your cycle. It really can be such an enlightening process! Once you start, it will take about three months to spot patterns and understand what your cycle consistently has in store for you.

Is there an app for that?

One way many women choose to track their menstrual cycle is by using an app. There are now hundreds of menstrual cycle tracking apps available, and the three of us often get asked which app we recommend. Our answer is less of a recommendation and more of a 'things to think about when you are choosing which app is best for you'.

There are three things we think are important to consider when choosing and using cycle-tracking apps.

1. History

   Does the app easily let you review your experience of previous months so that you can spot patterns over one, two or three months of data? Being able to look back over your cycle is important because this allows you to understand which physical and emotional symptoms are part of your cycle or to make connections with things that are going on in your life.

2. Advice

   Does the app try to offer you advice? Apps can be amazing for improving your understanding of the cycle and suggesting ways to alleviate symptoms, but before you start taking heed of said advice, check that the app you use is developed or recommended by experts. Even when apps say they have AI that 'learns' as you track, this might not be reliable. The app is learning only from what you are telling it, without context of what's happening inside your body, so it has to filter out how you feel because of your cycle and because of everything else that's going on in your life. This means it's almost impossible for an app's algorithm to be truly individualized to you and specifically to your menstrual cycle. Don't let the advice from an app override the signals your body is giving you, or your intuition about what your body needs. You are the expert on you.

3. Barrier

   Is the app acting as a barrier to important conversations? Apps that let you share your data with a trainer or your partner may seem like a great idea, but in practice, is this giving you an excuse to not talk about your cycle? Discussing your cycle is key to removing the mystery surrounding your physical and mental well-being.

Should I share?

Menstrual cycle data can feel like private, intimate information, and you don't have to share it if you don't want to. Just tuning in to your cycle holds the most value for you to improve your body literacy; it will build your confidence, improve your mental health and reduce your anxiety. Yet sharing this information is often useful. It gives those close to you, such as your partner, useful context for how you're feeling, so you don't have to cope with them asking why you're so moody, tired or quiet – they'll just understand that it's the time of your cycle, when you need a bit more space and grace.

If you use a massage therapist, it might also be useful to mention to them that you're on your period and, if this applies to you, are much more sensitive to touch and pain at this time. Similarly, you could tell your physio where you are in your cycle and ask them to include that information in your records, because the cycle can be the cause of joint pain or muscle tightness. You may ask your teammates to push you on in your CrossFit class if you're feeling low, or ask to take the lead in running club, because it's the time in your cycle when you feel awesome.

Tracking can also help your doctor diagnose any conditions you may be suffering from. The more information you can provide, the better, such as when your symptoms flare up and then settle, and what you were doing, eating, stressing about at the time; the time of your cycle, the season – all this insight can help your doctor identify and resolve the root cause of your health problems more quickly and efficiently.

Tracking, turned up a notch

We hope you're convinced that cycle tracking is a really important tool for allowing you to listen to what your body is telling you, so that you're more equipped to get the most out of your active life. If you're having significant challenges understanding your cycle, or why you are getting severe cycle symptoms, then taking a look 'under the hood' can be really insightful. For most women, in-depth tracking is not necessary, but there may be times when your cycle is impacting you and you really want to understand it more. Whether you're having bad symptoms or heavy periods, trying to get pregnant, lost your cycle altogether or you suspect that you're in the perimenopausal phase, this can help you and your doctor identify what's going on with your cycle.

In-depth tracking can include measurements such as body temperature.[13] Taken accurately, the consistent rise in body temperature on waking each morning can give a good insight into the length of your cycle phases and indicate that you have ovulated. If you want to know when in your cycle you are ovulating, you can also use ovulation test strips. You pee on these sticks daily about a week into your cycle, and the tests detect a surge in luteinizing hormone, which happens just before ovulation. You can get ovulation sticks that simply show a colour or a line when luteinizing hormone is high, or digital ones, which have a slightly more sophisticated display.

An exciting new technology that we work with closely is hormone monitoring via a saliva sample that you collect at home.[14] We're really excited by this as it means women can easily provide regular samples that give an individualized record of their hormones across the whole cycle. This detailed service can be the key to unlocking cycle symptoms or underlying cycle issues, because knowing the levels and balance of these hormones across your cycle can help you have a healthy cycle with manageable symptoms. This type of monitoring tool is also a good way to help understand why your periods have stopped, if used in conjunction with training and diet information. It allows you to confirm whether the menstrual cycle has been suppressed by energy deficiency or any other physical or emotional stress. Importantly, it also allows you to confirm whether the things you're doing to try to kick-start your menstrual cycle are succeeding. Just because your periods start again doesn't mean the whole cycle is healthy. Cycles can be infertile or dysfunctional even if your periods arrive back on the scene, since a truly healthy cycle contains both a period and ovulation, which ensure the hormones of the cycle ebb and flow in their predictable fashion. Only hormone monitoring can give you this kind of insight.

The point to any of these in-depth cycle tracking methods is that they enable an expert practitioner to interpret what you are finding and advise what action you can take.

What you might find

Once you start tracking, you'll notice lots of amazing things about how your cycle makes you feel, physically and emotionally. You may start to suss out exactly what's happening over the course of your cycle due to that wonderful hormone roller coaster.

The rise of awesome oestrogen

From the first day of your period, the follicular phase begins and your oestrogen starts to rise. Oestrogen has a lot of superpowers for active women because receptors for this hormone are found throughout the brain, in areas not only associated with reproduction, but also cognition and emotion. Oestrogen influences the production of serotonin, the 'good mood' hormone, and positivity, motivation and energy levels are high around the second week of the cycle. So, you might find your motivation to get up and go is greater in the first half of the cycle. Research has shown that in active women, motivation to train is highest around ovulation,[15] when oestrogen reaches its peak.[16] Some really interesting research, albeit in rodents rather than humans, has shown that oestrogen influences the desire to move.[17] In mice bred specifically not to produce oestrogen, sluggish behaviour was observed. When these mice were given a dose of oestrogen, this super-hormone caused them to explore, play and run further than they had before. While this research was not conducted on humans, given the fact that the mechanism for this change in behaviour under the influence of oestrogen is in an ancient part of the brain found in all mammals, it is plausible that the effect may hold true in humans too.

Since oestrogen helps us feel more sociable, when oestrogen is high you may find you enjoy working out in group sessions more or feel like you gel more with team dynamics. We also tend to be more emotionally resilient at this time of the cycle, so you may be more tolerant of an irritating partner or a difficult boss at this time. You may also be more open to constructive feedback, more capable of having difficult conversations or dealing with the mental load that largely falls on women.

Oestrogen can also make you feel more confident, competitive,[18] impulsive[19] and driven by reward. We once heard from a mountain-biker who felt that at this time of her cycle she found it much easier to hurl herself down the side of a steep hill, whereas later on in the cycle she felt more tentative. Feeling courageous is a great thing to tune in to, whether you want to use it to your advantage in sport or work, to plan or to take on new challenges in life.

Protective progesterone

After ovulation, you enter what we call the luteal phase, or second half of your cycle. Progesterone rises in this phase, and if oestrogen is your get-out-there-and-take-on-the-world hormone, progesterone is your be-calm-steady-Eddie hormone. Progesterone is actually the 'pro-gestation' hormone, as in it supports early pregnancy, and the behaviours it's trying to influence are to protect a newly implanted embryo – except most of the time there is no embryo, because we haven't conceived. But like oestrogen, progesterone does a whole lot more than help with getting and staying pregnant.

Among other things, progesterone soothes our central nervous system – think natural anti-anxiety medication.[20] Progesterone influences the neurotransmitter in the brain that helps promote calmness, good mood, and sleep. Sometimes active women frown when we tell them about progesterone, because calm and sleepy isn't the look they're going for. But progesterone isn't a sedative; its influence on the brain is positive, because it helps calm the circuits that can create a state of high anxiety, which isn't helpful for anyone. It has also been shown to reduce the sensation of pain.[21]

Feeling hot, hot, hot

One of the defining features of the second half of the cycle after ovulation is an increase in basal metabolic rate, or the amount of energy you use per day, which in turn increases body temperature by up to half a degree. If you accurately record your temperature on waking each morning, you will be able to see this rise in body temperature just after ovulation and throughout the second half of your cycle. It's how some women track their cycle and identify their fertile period when trying to get pregnant. Half a degree in body temperature doesn't sound like much, but our body temperature is tightly regulated. When we shiver or sweat, that's our body's way of making sure that our internal core temperature stays within a tight range to allow all our systems to work well. The rise in temperature in the second half of the cycle means that we tend to sweat more to keep our body temperature within this range, especially during exercise.[22] This means that while staying hydrated is always important, it's even more so in this part of your cycle.

The rise in metabolic rate also means you are burning more calories at this time of your cycle – about 150 calories extra per day. Research shows that women eat slightly more during this time of the cycle to compensate for this extra calorie burn.[23] But before you get excited and reach for a justified extra Hobnob, you don't need to actively seek out more food, since our brain instinctively makes us eat a bit more on each of those days.

A hormone hangover

Once progesterone and oestrogen have had their time to shine across the cycle, both hormones drop back to very low levels to end the cycle. This is known as the premenstrual phase, because it happens in the days before your next period starts. If the egg that was released at ovulation wasn't fertilized by a sperm, this 'unsuccessful' (in terms of pregnancy) cycle comes to an end. Far from being 'hormonal' during this time, women are actually experiencing a withdrawal from the influence of the amazing hormones that have been at high levels in the previous phase of the cycle. It's like a hormone hangover, if you will: you've been bathed in the awesomeness of oestrogen and its influence on good mood, and in progesterone with its calming, anti-anxiety effects, and then they are taken away, and that's what causes many of the negative symptoms – all 150 of them that have been described by women at this premenstrual time of their cycle.

Keeping us going, growing and glowing

While understanding our experience of our cycle is about recognizing how oestrogen and progesterone can affect how we feel, physically and emotionally, from day to day or week to week across the cycle, we could not leave out how important these hormones are for our overall and long-term health. Every time these hormones rise across the cycle, it's like a deposit into our health bank. For example, oestrogen is important for building bone density, maintaining cardiovascular health, boosting our immune function and helping our muscles repair and grow (provided we exercise them!). Progesterone's health benefits reach to breast, cardiovascular and nervous-system health, as well as cognitive function.[24] It's this range of roles our menstrual cycle hormones play, beyond affecting our ability to reproduce, that makes our cycle such a powerful influence on our health and well-being across every area of our lives.

Step 3: Symptoms and what to do about them

Don't suffer in cycles

In a survey of over 14,000 active women by online training platform Strava and menstrual cycle app FitrWoman, 88% said that their cycle symptoms impacted negatively on their training at some point of their cycle.[25] And no matter what group of women we are working with, from fifteen-year-old school students to elite footballers to midlife running-clubbers, the outcome is the same: most of them have some days (for some, it's whole weeks) of the cycle where they can't be who they want to be because symptoms of their cycle are holding them back.

The common thread among all these women isn't just that their cycle is impacting their life and their ability to exercise, but that they have simply accepted that to be their lot. Many have accepted that symptoms are just 'part of being a woman' without trying to make them better, while others have tried a couple of things but then felt embarrassed to go back to the doctor, or even explore other practitioners, because they don't want to be seen as fragile or moaning.

If we switched this scenario and replaced menstrual cycle issues with a lower back issue that flares up regularly, is painful, affects your work, your motivation and your ability to exercise and even, on the days where the pain gets you down, gets in the way of your relationships, the outcome is likely to be different. You will probably have spoken to several people about your back pain. You will have tried to figure out what type of treatment you need to stop it flaring up, and when it does, what you need to do. You've probably visited your doctor, a physio or other experts to find the right approach, and diligently tried the strategies they suggested to establish an approach that ensures your back injury rarely bothers you. When it does, you've taken advice about stretching and strapping techniques you can use, and pain relief cream you can apply, that seem to keep the interruption to a minimum, without doing your back any more damage.

It should be the same approach with our menstrual cycle. We should be happy to diligently explore strategies until we find the right one. But too often, when it comes to issues related to women's health, we don't give it the same attitude and attention we would for less intimate issues.

The pillars of good health

Before we go into the detail of evidence-based strategies for managing cycle symptoms, we want to stress that getting the basic pillars of health in good shape will really help any negative symptoms of your cycle. These are sleep, exercise, diet and stress management. There's a lot of research to support the fact that if you get enough sleep, your diet is balanced and full of nutritious food, delivered to your body at the right time, you exercise regularly and you find ways to manage stress that work for you, your overall health will benefit.

This is entirely true for your hormone health as well, and your hormone health is fundamentally important for a healthy menstrual cycle – one that isn't painful or that doesn't involve symptoms that aren't manageable. We encourage you to take a look at those important pillars first. There might be something in your diet or lifestyle that you notice triggers or worsens symptoms, or when your cycle symptoms are milder there might be something about your exercise routine or your work that is different at that time. Cycle tracking is a really good way for you to make those connections.

> **Bella**
> Medication can often be a quick fix for something that can and should be managed by diet and lifestyle instead. When it comes to menstrual health, it's easy for

doctors like me to prescribe something like the pill, when in reality some patients could adjust some lifestyle factors and see an equivalent benefit to cycle symptoms. There's no doubt it's harder to do it that way, but often all someone needs is a nudge in the right direction; someone to draw attention to the amount of stress that person is under without making time for self-care, or that their relationship with alcohol or exercise might be excessive. With the right support and advice, some simple (but not always easy!) changes to how we go about our lives can have profound effects on our health and well-being.

Pandemic cycles

It's easy for us to tell you that lifestyle, diet, exercise and stress play a big role in your experience of the cycle, but much harder for you to make changes to those things as part of your cycle strategy. Sometimes women want to know what magic supplement they can take, without addressing a diet that isn't balanced or the lack of self-care that underpins high stress levels. But something Covid-19 gave us (in the midst of all it took away) was a perfect experiment to show how these things really do impact our menstrual cycles.

A study of Australian Olympic athletes in 2020 showed how their menstrual cycles had been affected by a less intense, less pressured phase of home training instead of their usual routine of competitive events and the Olympic Games.[26] It was in one sense a more relaxed spell for elite athletes, yet simultaneously a highly stressful time, full of uncertainty, as it was for us all. In the study, female athletes shared how their cycles had changed under these circumstances, from having heavier periods, infrequent periods or getting periods back after some time without having had them at all. This natural experiment showed how changes in diet, training, recovery and stress impacted the characteristics of women's periods and cycles.

In 2015, the American College of Obstetricians and Gynecologists made a recommendation that at every visit, healthcare professionals should ask about a woman's menstrual cycle. That's because when a woman is generally healthy, her menstrual cycle will go smoothly and will include both ovulation and a period with very few, or at least manageable, symptoms. When she is unhealthy in some way, her cycle is likely to reflect that. A recent research study of nearly 80,000 women showed that having an irregular and long menstrual cycle was associated with a greater risk of premature death (defined as dying before you get to seventy years).[27] Since your lifestyle has the potential to impact your menstrual cycle hormones, if your diet is poor, you aren't managing stress, you aren't getting enough sleep, you smoke, you're underweight or overweight, don't exercise enough or exercise too much, then your cycle characteristics can reflect these factors.

Menstrual cycle symptom-busters

If your cycle symptoms are getting in the way of you doing what you want to do with your life, then get curious about what might make things better. In women whose symptoms are really debilitating, more support from healthcare professionals might also be needed. Pain or other symptoms that are anything but mild and manageable shouldn't be part of a healthy cycle and it's important to seek medical support and diligently explore strategies and solutions until you find something that works.

Period pain

Period pain is common and is usually experienced as cramps that come on each cycle just before or at the time bleeding begins. These cramps typically last about one to three days.

They may start as strong and reduce as the hours pass, or they may come and go more randomly. Once again, every woman's experience of period pain will differ, and cramps can range from barely noticeable through to severe. In younger women, periods can be more painful during the first couple of years after the first menstruation but usually improve after the age of twenty.

> ### Emma
>
> On her ninetieth birthday, I visited my grandmother-in-law and we started talking about how much things had changed in her lifetime. She said that as a young woman she would get excruciating periods, but that at that time, even if you did go to the doctor – which most women wouldn't – doctors would say it was normal and advise you to just get on with it. Even though things have changed greatly for women and their health since she was a young woman in the 1940s, perhaps they haven't improved as much as we'd like to think. That very same week, following a menstrual cycle workshop, I spoke to a woman who loved to exercise and compete but was floored by period pain every month. And when she said 'floored', she meant it – as in, curled up under her desk at work. When I asked her whether anyone at work had noticed, she replied: 'I was under the desk, so no one even saw.'
>
> I asked her what she had tried so far to address the symptoms and she said she'd been to a couple of doctors, one of whom told her it was normal, while the other offered the pill as her only option. In the end, she didn't make any progress in getting relief from her symptoms. There she was, a young woman in 2020, in a similar situation to my grandmother-in-law in 1945. While there isn't a single quick

fix for period pain for everyone, severe pain isn't normal and there are many options listed below to improve this symptom.

Proactive painkilling

Period pain is usually caused by prostaglandins, chemicals released by the body in order to have a healthy period. Although these inflammatory chemicals are a necessary part of the process, they can cause the blood vessels and the muscles of the uterus to contract too strongly, which causes pain. They are also often the cause of the upset tummy that some women experience around the time of their period. The level of prostaglandins is often highest on the first day of your period, so the pain and tummy upset might be worse at this time. To manage period pain, ibuprofen or other non-steroidal anti-inflammatory drugs like aspirin (NSAID) work by preventing excess prostaglandins being produced.[28] The key here is to not wait until you're doubled over before taking the pain relief. Start on the recommended dose before you even get period pain (but you know it's coming, perhaps by your tracking or feeling a dull ache in your tummy) and take it at the recommended frequency throughout the time you usually experience pain. If you've tried taking painkillers before without success, you may find this proactive approach works. Ibuprofen and other NSAIDs can also significantly lighten your flow when taken during bleeding days, making your period more manageable if it's usually heavy.[29]

Wonderful warmth

Heat is a great period pain reliever and there's research to show that heat packs are as effective as painkillers for alleviating period pain in some women, especially if used in conjunction with painkillers. Whether you pop a hot-water bottle on your tummy as you drive to the gym or put an adhesive heat pack under your shirt during your work commute, heat is a versatile and easy-to-use strategy.

Ancient analgesics

Yoga has been shown to be effective at reducing period pain when performed regularly across the cycle – thirty minutes twice a week – and at the time when period pain occurs.[30] Yoga poses can help improve blood flow to the abdomen, counteracting the constriction of blood flow that results from the contractions in the uterus. Adding yoga into your schedule might alleviate symptoms enough to allow you to enjoy your regular training or be a useful pain reliever before bed. Yoga will have other benefits, including stress management, which could also pay off on your hormonal health.

Many active people use acupuncture to relieve aches and pains, and this can extend to period pain; research has shown acupuncture to be effective in alleviating inflammation,[31] which is great news for managing cycle symptoms because we know that inflammation can make these worse.

Micronutrients

Some important micronutrients in our food have been shown to alleviate period pain, so you can use your diet as an effective way to help with symptoms, in any of the following ways.

- Eat foods rich in magnesium and zinc in the lead-up to and throughout your period – well, always, really, given how awesome they are, but particularly at this time, as research has shown these minerals help reduce the amount of prostaglandins you produce and their associated side effect of pain and cramping.[32] Because magnesium works so quickly, you can try supplementing just during your period.[33]

- Incorporate more oily fish into your diet or take some fish oil supplements: fish oil has been found to reduce period pain by 30% after being taken for two months.[34] The amazing omega-3s in fish oil have an anti-inflammatory effect and reduce the level of prostaglandins.

- Consider cutting dairy from your diet. There is no robust research that supports this finding yet, but menstrual health practitioners have seen this strategy to be effective with so many of their patients that it's worth considering. The problem with dairy is that a protein called A1 casein can, in some people, cause an inflammatory response in the body by disrupting the immune system.[35] This disruption can cause symptoms such as hay fever, sinus infections, eczema and asthma, but women may also see this A1 casein intolerance manifest as menstrual cycle problems such as period pain, acne, PMS and heavy periods. If you suspect that you may have a problem with cow's dairy, then omit it from your diet for about three months to see if that's the case. You can substitute non-dairy alternatives such as almond, oat, soy, rice or coconut milk. You can also continue to have sheep and goat dairy as they don't contain A1 casein. Do remember that if you cut out dairy then you are at risk of becoming deficient in calcium, so make sure you get enough of this important micronutrient.

- Stay hydrated. Hydration is basic but vital, particularly throughout your period, when your menstrual blood loss can contribute to dehydration, which in turn can cause headaches. Try to sip on water regularly throughout the day, checking that when you pee, your urine is a pale straw colour. If it's much darker, start to increase your water intake – but not in one big down-a-pint-of-water style, as that's a really ineffective hydration strategy, as most of it will end up being peed out before it has been absorbed.

- Try turmeric: the active ingredient in turmeric, called curcumin, is an effective anti-inflammatory that helps combat period pain[36] and endometriosis.[37] Either incorporate it into your diet by cooking with turmeric (it's excellent in curries) or take a supplement after eating when it can be more readily absorbed.

A powerful pill

We can't talk about relieving cycle symptoms without including hormonal contraception. It's one of the most commonly prescribed solutions for active women who suffer from period pain and other cycle symptoms that interfere with their active lives. Clinical trials show that up to 80% of women find pain relief from significant period pain after starting the pill.[38] Alternatively, a hormonal contraceptive coil can be inserted into your uterus by a nurse. This releases progestin over a five-year period which acts as a contraceptive but is often also prescribed to lighten periods and to manage period pain, particularly the severe kind related to endometriosis.

Premenstrual syndrome (PMS)

Although there are many symptoms that can be attributed to PMS, the most commonly reported are headaches, breast pain, gastrointestinal issues, anxiety, brain fog, and difficulty sleeping.[39] For many women, experiencing emotional, physical and behavioural premenstrual symptoms is a normal part of the cycle, and for most these symptoms are manageable. However, for some women these become so significant that they can interfere with daily life.

If that's the case, then you might be experiencing premenstrual syndrome (PMS)[40] or premenstrual dysphoric disorder (PMDD),[41] each of which have their own medical diagnosis. While about eight in ten women say they experience one or more premenstrual symptoms, about three in ten women experience symptoms significant enough to warrant a clinical diagnosis of PMS and about 8% of them suffer from PMDD, which is a type of severe PMS associated with psychiatric symptoms.[42]

Sadly, too many women suffer in silence and just put up with the symptoms that occur in the days before their period, even though they affect them significantly. Whether you have a clinical diagnosis of PMS or you just notice that you have physical or emotional changes that crop up in the days before your period, it's possible that there are things that can help.

The first step to managing PMS is to track your cycle so you know what symptoms you're dealing with. For example, there can be triggers in your diet that make symptoms worse, such as caffeine, alcohol or highly processed foods. Cycle tracking can really help tease out what is sending your symptoms into over-drive. There are also foods that can help alleviate symptoms because they have anti-inflammatory properties or support a healthy hormone balance, which we'll talk about in Chapter 8 where we focus on female-centric nutrition.

Exercise can also help premenstrual symptoms in the short term – because the endorphins released by exercising are natural mood elevators and painkillers – and in the long term – women who exercise regularly have been shown to have fewer symp-toms.[43] Even if you don't feel like exercising when symptoms are at their worst, if you can find some type of physical activity that you can manage, even if it's just walking, it's almost certain to help your physical or emotional symptoms at this time. The important thing is finding what works for you.

Warning: Contents may be emotionally fragile

Premenstrual symptoms can often impact mood and emotion. Even if the symptoms are mild and don't need treatment as clin-ical PMS, they can still get in the way of your active lifestyle. From affecting your confidence, your motivation to exercise, your rela-tionships with your trainer, workmates, partner or family – if you are emotionally fragile at this time, it's important to acknowledge that and devise a plan that helps. It should be very individual to you and your needs. It could be that the type of exercise you do on these days changes to reflect your mood; if you feel angry or frustrated at this time, maybe some hardcore sessions will do the trick. If your mood is low, what exercise or training session really gives you a buzz?[44] What music can you listen to that might help? Research has shown that exercising, listening to music, seeking social support and engaging in positive self-talk can all help manage low mood.[45]

In a team or group setting, whether that's at work or when you're working out or doing sport, knowing that your mood or emotions change in the premenstrual phase is an important thing to notice and talk about. We've seen dynamics severely affected because one person in a team had PMS symptoms that made her less tolerant of her fellow teammates. But because she didn't say anything, and nor did anyone else, every month there were a few days of total upheaval in the team as people tiptoed around her, resented her, were frustrated by her being equally frustrated by them, and the whole atmosphere went to pot. No matter how talented that team was, their lack of cohesion and connection affected their performance.

When it comes to premenstrual emotions, it's important to remember that timing is everything. If you get premenstrual mood symptoms, rather than trying to talk about it in the heat of the moment, it's often helpful to wait until a week or so later, when you're back in the fist-pumping part of your cycle, and you can have an emotionally resilient discussion about what people can expect and what would help during the premenstrual part of your cycle. At this time, when you aren't caught up in what you're feeling, there's a better chance of working out a strategy with your team, trainer, boss or colleagues. It might be changing the communication style during those days, such as how feedback is delivered, or simply that knowing what's going on allows those around you to support you better.

Don't crash and burn

There is evidence that in the second half of the cycle, as progesterone levels increase, we become slightly more insulin resistant,[46] which means insulin – which is responsible for keeping our blood-sugar level stable – becomes less effective. This can lead to spikes and crashes of blood sugar, which don't feel great. When our blood sugar is slightly less stable, this can also cause food cravings or periods of low energy. It's worth noticing, through cycle tracking, whether there are certain times of the cycle when it feels harder to maintain an even keel when it comes to energy and appetite. In the second half of the cycle it might be necessary to really focus on eating low-glycaemic-index foods – which release their energy more slowly and avoid sugar spikes in our blood – such as vegetables, beans and lentils, rather than pasta or bread. It's also useful to eat regularly, not leaving too long between snacks and meals. This approach to 'fuelling' can be the difference between getting your energy levels right throughout the day to help you focus at work or nail your workout session.

Tummy trouble

Gastrointestinal issues can be a big problem for women during the premenstrual phase or as your period starts. Constipation can happen because the peaking progesterone during the second half of your cycle has slowed down transit time through your digestive tract. This means your body has a chance to extract more water from faecal material as it moves through, and this leads to poos which are hard to pass. If you find bloating or constipation a problem, then stay extra diligent about keeping on top of your hydration and get plenty of fibre in your diet too.

At the other end of this gastro spectrum, other women will experience diarrhoea around the time of their period. The same chemicals that caused our period pain – prostaglandins – are also often the cause of this upset tummy. Just as we use them for period pain, aspirin and ibuprofen help block the production of prostaglandins and lower their levels, which helps alleviate these symptoms.[47] Since both can irritate the digestive tract (aspirin more so than ibuprofen), it's worth trying to find tablets with a gastro-resistant coating, which are a bit kinder on your tummy.

Heavy menstrual bleeding

Although there is a clinical definition for heavy menstrual bleeding, which is losing over 80ml of blood during a period, in reality, who measures the quantity of their menstrual blood? No one we know. For most women, whether a period is heavy or not depends more on how well you're able to manage your flow. If you're changing period products every couple of hours or sooner, or doubling up on tampons and pads, it's likely you have a heavy flow. You might also call it heavy bleeding if your flow is normal but the length of your period is longer than normal – eight days or more.

About 40% of women have heavy periods,[48] and while most just learn to cope with heavy bleeding, it brings with it both physical and emotional challenges. Women with heavy periods can have increased anxiety over managing their period, fear of leaking and continually worrying where the nearest bathroom might be to change products. Health-wise, heavy periods put you at an increased risk of iron-deficiency anaemia. If you're someone who is very sporty, heavy periods may also have a performance implication, with one study showing that marathon runners who reported heavy periods also registered slower times.[49] Although this doesn't rule out other factors that might have been responsible for the difference, the researchers suggested that iron deficiency could be responsible.

Active women are naturally at a greater risk of iron deficiency. This is because high-impact exercise, such as running, ruptures red blood cells in the feet, which contain the iron (the posh name is foot-strike haemolysis).[50] Added to that, inflammation caused by exercise (which is part of the inherent recovery process that occurs when exercising) reduces the amount of iron we can absorb from our diet. Factor in heavy periods, when both the menstrual blood you're losing contains iron and your natural ability to absorb iron is reduced through the increased levels of inflammation brought on by having your period, and you can see why active women with heavy periods are at a real risk of developing iron deficiency. It's a quadruple-whammy.

Symptoms of iron deficiency include fatigue, breathlessness and light-headedness. If you think you might be on the low side for iron, don't start taking supplements before getting your levels checked with a blood test by your doctor. Taking supplemental iron when you don't need to can have equally disruptive side effects, such as constipation, nausea and stomach pain (iron supplements taken in liquid form are often easier on the digestive tract). Dr Bella often advises her patients who are taking iron supplement pills or liquids to drink these with orange juice, as vitamin C helps with its absorption.

Lighten the flow

A heavy flow is often caused by a hormonal imbalance (in particular high oestrogen and/or low progesterone), which can be brought on by a range of things, including inadequate diet or sleep, or by stress. Good gut health is key to preventing high oestrogen because healthy gut bacteria escort oestrogen safely out of your body, whereas unhealthy gut bacteria can reactivate oestrogen and cause it to be reabsorbed back into your body. Exercise in general is excellent for gut health, and also allows excess oestrogen to leave the body via sweat. Taking ibuprofen or other NSAIDs, or having a hormonal contraceptive coil inserted, are also effective ways of lightening your flow.

Not the best time for breasts

Just before your period each cycle, your breasts may become enlarged or sore.[51] They may also become lumpy, so first know what's normal for you, so that you can detect any abnormal lumps and bumps should they present themselves. In the 70% of women who experience breast pain as part of their menstrual cycle, about 20% would describe the pain as moderate to extreme.[52] Emma's research in athletes showed that in the women who reported breast pain, 70% said it was related to their cycle. However, women don't usually wear a different bra at this time of the cycle, when their breasts change size or shape, so make sure you try adjusting your usual bra to accommodate that. We've dedicated the whole of Chapter 6 to the art and science of breast support, but – spoiler alert – a well-fitting bra can help alleviate pain and discomfort – like letting your belt out a notch after a big holiday meal! If your breast changes throughout the cycle really compromise the fit of your usual bra, then it may even be worth getting one that fits well just during those few days of the cycle when things are different from your norm.

Premenstrual magnification

Some symptoms aren't actually symptoms of the cycle at all, but a worsening of symptoms that are due to another underlying cause and generally experienced at the end of the cycle.[53] Headaches in particular, particularly migraines, have been linked to this phase of the cycle, with 50% of female migraine sufferers experiencing a worsening of these types of headaches just before their period.[54] This premenstrual worsening of symptoms that you tend to experience all the time – such as irritable bowel syndrome (IBS),[55] mood disturbance[56] or acne, as well as headaches – is called premenstrual magnification.[57] Rather than treat them as PMS symptoms, you need to get to the underlying conditions and treat those.

Emma

I have first-hand experience of premenstrual magnification. As an IBS sufferer, I am used to its symptoms, but have never understood their inconsistency. I was forever trying to find things that triggered the painful spasms and unbearable bloating, so I could eliminate them from my diet. When I started tracking my cycle, things suddenly fell into place. There were certain times of my cycle, the premenstrual phase in particular, where my IBS was indeed very irritable, and triggered further by lots of things that usually didn't cause me a problem. With that knowledge, I knew to be especially diligent about not doing anything at that time that would risk bringing on my IBS symptoms, like going too long without eating or having too much caffeine.

Habit cues that help

Habit cues enable you to recognize when a particular part of your cycle is coming up and to know what it's going to throw at you. Maybe you feel it physically or emotionally, or you know what to expect based on your tracking, and that's your cue to do something that will help get the most out of the next few hours or days. It may be that you use your premenstrual symptoms as a cue to be proactive about pain management, because you would otherwise suffer badly from period pain. Or perhaps after your period finishes, you always feel amazing for the following week, and so your period ending is your cue to go out there and take advantage of that wonderful oestrogen-fuelled physiology.

Knowing what your cycle feels like can help you create an energy plan across the whole month. When are the times that you need to do things that give you energy and make you feel better? That might be a restorative type of exercise, like yoga, but it might also be baking or listening to a certain type of music. Whatever it looks like for you, anticipating what your cycle is about to bring, and being able to be proactive about it, will develop your cycle resilience. Develop habit cues. What are the cues your body is giving you to start or stop doing something, so that you can prevent symptoms from happening or exploit the positive parts of your cycle?

Don't suffer in silence

Symptoms related to your cycle can sometimes be down to underlying conditions such as endometriosis, a condition characterized by severe inflammation and pain around the time of your period. These symptoms can impact your physical, sexual and mental health, and shockingly, it can take up to eight years for some women to be diagnosed.[58]

One of the most common cycle dysfunctions that we come across is polycystic ovarian syndrome (PCOS). It's actually the most common endocrine disorder, affecting 7% of women of reproductive age.[59] PCOS isn't about one symptom alone, like cysts on ovaries, but a set of symptoms, including anovulatory cycles (where ovulation doesn't happen during the menstrual cycle) and an excess of androgen hormones (like testosterone), which causes symptoms such as acne, excess body hair, hair loss and weight gain.[60]

Whether they have an underlying condition or not, women tell us all the time about how they haven't been able to get the support they need for physical or emotional suffering related to their cycle. Give yourself the best chance of getting the right help by tracking your cycle and arming yourself with as much insight as possible into what's happening with your body. The bottom line is that if your cycle symptoms affect your day-to-day life, then you shouldn't hold back from seeking help from your doctor. If you feel your symptoms aren't being acknowledged appropriately or you feel you are being fobbed off, then don't give up, and seek medical advice from a different doctor.

Step 4: Training around your cycle

One of the most empowering things we can share with you is that, with a healthy cycle, your capacity to perform is not limited by the ebb and flow of your hormonal rhythm. You can channel your inner champion any day of the month. There is evidence that fitness and performance metrics such as aerobic fitness, strength, power or speed are unaffected by the hormonal fluctuation of your cycle,[61] and neither are cognitive capability and intelligence.[62]

But just because your body has the capacity to perform well, it doesn't mean that you're always going to feel like it, or that your cycle won't put some challenges in your way to trip you up. It's no good being in the best shape of your life to run a PB at the parkrun if you're doubled over with period pain. Nor can you expect to access the speed and power you're capable of if you feel bloated and sluggish. The way hormones influence things like mood, metabolism and motivation means that the strategies you need to adopt to get the best out of yourself may have to change on different days of your cycle. What or when you eat, how much sleep you need, how you manage anxiety, and how you prepare and recover from training, may need to vary from day to day to cope with the changing physiology of the cycle. If you tune in to your cycle experience and recognize when it's a superpower and what you need to do to overcome its challenging symptoms, then every day can be a podium finish. Instead of becoming a self-fulfilling prophecy – 'I always miss my shots at goal at this time of my cycle' or 'My coordination is affected by my cycle' – the narrative could be 'What do I have to do differently to prepare for goal-shooting on the days of my cycle when I feel a bit clumsy?' or 'How can I be kinder to myself when I don't play so well on those days, because I know that I'm usually pretty good and I'm proud that I showed up and did my best.'

A universal template for training?

One of the first things athletes and coaches ask us is how to train around the cycle, and we know they're hoping that we'll hand over 'the plan'. We then have to slow the conversation down and explain that, first, every woman's experience of her cycle will be different, and the 'plan' will have to be unique to her. Second, the foundations of health, fitness and peak performance come from doing the first three stages of this chapter well: gaining the knowledge, tracking and understanding the cycle, and managing its symptoms. Training in sync with your cycle is the cherry on the cake – it's not the be all and end all, and certainly not something to get obsessed with. Yet it can be a really brilliant way to feel like you're working with your body, not against it.

Oestrogen loves high-intensity training

Metabolism is the process our body uses to turn what we eat and drink into the energy we need to function. Our metabolism is influenced by the phases of the cycle, and research suggests that our body is better at different times of the cycle from others at using carbohydrates or fats to fuel our exercise.[63]

In the follicular phase of the cycle, generally the second week, when oestrogen is high, more glucose (a carbohydrate) is transported into our muscle fibres, to be used as energy, and research suggests this can improve our ability to perform high-intensity training as this relies on carbohydrates, which give us energy quickly, as the main fuel.[64] So, for some women, high-intensity exercise might feel really good during this phase of the cycle. Fats take longer to convert into energy so they can't provide the energy needed for high-intensity exercise. Women's greater fat stores make our bodies really good at sustaining lower-intensity, longer-duration exercise.

Because your body is particularly good at using carbohydrates in the first half of the cycle, if you're doing longer training sessions, you'll need to actively keep your energy topped up as your body is burning through those carbs. This means ensuring you arrive at the start of training well-fuelled by having had a carbohydrate-rich meal or snack about an hour before you train and even having a mid-training snack at an appropriate moment to top up your energy levels.

Rockin' that recovery

Oestrogen is at it again when it comes to recovery: it is our friend with benefits. Oestrogen improves muscle repair and regeneration through the activation and multiplication of satellite cells – cells which can develop into skeletal muscle cells, which are essential in helping muscles repair after the inevitable damage that happens as part of hard training, or performing movements which are unfamiliar, known as microtrauma. Oestrogen also has antioxidant effects, which reduce the muscle damage caused by your workouts. All of this means that the recovery process after exercise is more efficient during this first half of our cycle.

You may be familiar with DOMS – delayed onset of muscle soreness – which happens after you complete a new or challenging workout. DOMS is the painful sensation in the muscles you've exercised that hits the next day and sometimes even intensifies the day after that. The pain is an indication of the microtrauma, or damage, that has occurred in your muscles through the exercise. Although it doesn't feel great, it's a sign that the body is recovering from this experience, that you're adapting to your training, and getting stronger and fitter. Researchers have found that oestrogen might protect us from suffering such muscle damage after exercise. When a marker in the blood that indicates muscle damage was measured, the levels were found to be lower at the time of the cycle when oestrogen is highest.[65] So in this first, or follicular phase, the awesomeness of oestrogen is helping your muscles recover better.

Tuning in to your cycle can help you notice how your body responds to certain workouts at different times. Do you recover more quickly at particular points in your cycle, or have less soreness after a particular training session, whether that's an intense HIIT session or a long training run? If you understand the reasons behind this, you can start to get more out of your training because in the first part of your cycle you can leave less recovery time between hard sessions or schedule sessions in a different way to take advantage of how you feel after each one. Be sure to tune in to your own cycle to see how you feel; don't just take our word for it. Your body will tell you how quickly you're recovering and how ready you are to train again. Listen to it – because not allowing enough recovery between sessions and not fuelling that training and recovery properly can cause illness and injury.[66]

SSTiF training

With oestrogen giving us the edge during high-intensity workouts and helping us to recover better from them, researchers have been curious about whether these effects could be used to get more out of our training programme. While there have been only a couple of studies dedicated to this question at the time of writing, their findings have been consistent: if you do more strength or resistance training sessions in the follicular phase – the first half of your cycle – and don't do as many in the luteal phase – the second half of your cycle – you achieve greater gains in strength and muscle size, compared with spacing those training sessions evenly across your cycle.[67] The three of us call this 'Stacking Strength Training in Follicular' – or SSTiF – training. It's pretty revolutionary to use the physiology of your cycle to amplify the effects of your training; in fact, tracking your cycle and using that insight to train smarter and better is revolutionary, full stop – but SSTiF training takes it up a notch.

Specifically, SSTiF training research showed that when strength-training sessions occurred on every second day, or eight times, in the first half of the cycle, and once per week, or two times, during the second half of the cycle, versus spreading sessions out evenly across the weeks or condensing more sessions into the second half, the gains were greater. And we're not talking trivial effects: in one study, maximal strength increased by 40% when training was performed more frequently in the follicular phase and less frequently in the luteal phase, compared with a 27% increase in strength when that pattern was flipped.[68] Another study comparing stacking training in the follicular phase with training that was done every three days consistently across the cycle showed that maximal leg-strength improved over 30% in the follicular phase training versus 13% in the regularly spaced training programme.[69] In both those studies, the cross-sectional area of the muscles – that's how big they were – increased more in the SSTiF training regimes. So, if you tend to do eight to twelve strength sessions a month, stick three quarters of them in the first couple of weeks of your cycle and see how it goes; there's a chance you'll see greater adaptation and, even in a worst-case scenario, the research suggests, you'll see the same gains you would if you hadn't stacked your training in the follicular phase; so if you have the flexibility in your programme, it might be worth playing around with your training schedule to see if this approach suits you.

Of course, if you're fitting in higher-intensity training in the first half of your cycle, you'll need to accompany that with good rest and recovery – when the magic happens in terms of adaptation – and you'll have to be on top of your nutrition to support your body's repair and growth. As women, we need more protein post-exercise than men, and we need it, in combination with carbohydrate, within thirty minutes of finishing our workout.[70] This is the window of opportunity to refuel for optimum recovery. In this time frame your muscles can quickly absorb the nutrients you're putting in. The longer you leave it, the less successfully you will refuel your tired muscles. Get carbs and protein in after a workout and you restock your muscles with what they need to repair, grow and reduce muscle damage.[71] Thirty minutes isn't long once you've talked to your teammates, had a shower and prepared your food. The only way Baz could hit this window when she was training as a rower was to prep her food in advance and leave it on her boat rack so it was there as soon as she came off the water. It meant that, despite the fact her coach liked a lengthy debrief, she always hit her window of opportunity for refuelling. Remember that if you get recovery and nutrition wrong – particularly if you are SSTiF training – you could risk injury or illness, so make sure that if you're playing around with your training planning that you consider all of its elements, and not just one in isolation.

As with any training programme, SSTiF training won't generate the same response in all women – there is always a natural distribution of responses to training regimes. Lots of people cluster around the mean and show average improvements; some people adapt more, and some less than that. We also know that not everyone has the flexibility in their training programme to schedule different sessions according to their own individual cycle, but we think it's exciting to know that for this first half of the cycle, your physiology really is on your side as an active woman. That should feel like a superpower, so let your superhero cape flutter proudly during this time.

Loosen up!

Oestrogen has had a fairly good score card so far, what with all the good moods, motivation to train and better recovery. However, while its ability to help build and regenerate muscle may be protective against muscle injury, it has a detrimental effect on collagen, the main component of connective tissues such as ligaments and tendons. Research suggests oestrogen causes collagen to become more elastic which could be a risk factor for joint injury by increasing joint laxity – the looseness of the joint.[72] So while men's laxity remains constant over time, in women, laxity increases by about 5mm in the late follicular phase, when oestrogen is high. Some research suggests that for every 1.3mm increase in the laxity of our knee joints, the risk of anterior cruciate ligament (ACL) injury goes up four-fold.[73]

However, before anyone starts wearing knee braces and bubble wrap for this week of their cycle, increased injury risk is not just about having high oestrogen. Women don't fall over with every menstrual cycle, literally 'weak at the knees'. Injury is complex and is a culmination of risk factors, of which fluctuating oestrogen levels is just one. So instead of assuming you're more likely to get injured just before ovulation, tune in to your personal experience of the cycle. We've worked with active women who have recurrent niggles that sometimes flare up, such as a sore lower back or a tight hamstring. A physiotherapist may be busy looking for some musculoskeletal cause for the injury, but when the woman starts tracking the flare-ups alongside her menstrual cycle, this can show that they're happening at the same time within her cycle. A slight change in joint laxity around the pelvis can cause tilting that puts muscles slightly out of balance and results in back or hamstring niggles that quieten down after a few days. If you have an injury that flares up at this time of the cycle, this provides a powerful insight that can make you proactive about managing it. Perhaps you can tape the muscle or joint more diligently at that time or have more soft-tissue massage or ensure that your warm-up is more comprehensive. Tuning in to your cycle and knowing what's going on for you gives you the power to do something about it.

Calamity Jane

In the second half of the cycle, progesterone may be responsible for a slight change to your skill and coordination. This concept was introduced to Emma during a conversation with a hockey coach who said he could tell when certain players on his team were in this phase of their cycle because of how they played on the pitch. He noticed that a few of the women would have times when they were slightly off in their ability to deliver skill under pressure, to anticipate the movement of the game as well as other players around them, and it would always turn out that they were in this part of their cycle. Another coach mentioned how an archer would be slightly off in her feel for the bow. Both coaches used the same term 'slightly off' – nothing major, but just a disturbance in what is otherwise a consistent and finely tuned performance. There's not much research at all about the impact of progesterone on performance in skill-based sports, but research has shown that it may be related to progesterone's effect on the brain.[74] The key is to tune in to how you are influenced by your cycle. If you have a certain time of the month that you find you might be more clumsy or less coordinated, and it's a consistent observation in your cycle, then you can start to do something about it.

You might find this is improved by caffeine,[75] as it can influence alertness and cognition, or by aerobic exercise, which can enhance the signalling in your brain,[76] or by adding a session into your warm-up that fires up your neuromuscular system. Activities that involve strong muscle contractions, skill or agility can be particularly useful.[77] If you know your cycle affects your coordination and you've got a big tournament or event that falls at this time, you could start to plan competition day with some purpose, building in some caffeine to your pre-event snack and modifying your warm-up to include more aerobic work and drills that fire up your nervous system.

Squad goals

Once we've told coaches that there is no universal blueprint for training across the cycle, their next question is 'How on earth do

I organize training around the cycle when I'm working with a squad of thirty?' It's unrealistic to think that in a squad setting you'll be able to start organizing strength training around the first half of the cycle and tailoring individual schedules to individual cycles. That would be insanity! In these squad situations, we've seen coaches use a top-up set of strength training for athletes who are in their follicular phase and who feel like they can take on more and recover well at this time of their cycle. We love the term used by the Jennis fitness platform we work with: 'follicular finisher' – for when you're in that phase of your cycle and your prescribed training just isn't enough!

The bottom line when you're in a team setting and trying to work around everyone's cycles is to encourage everyone to use their own insight from their cycle tracking to (a) help them anticipate and proactively manage their own cycle symptoms, which means they show up being able to give their best, and (b) to know when the time is right to do a real beast of a session. This personal insight and action can be done by each individual so they each get the best out of themselves on any given day. One athlete might arrive at training having done fifteen minutes of yoga before she left because she knows this is an excellent strategy to manage period pain, another might have listened to a specific type of music on the way to training to help energize herself, another might be avoiding caffeine because she knows that triggers her symptoms, while another is drinking a coffee before training because she knows it mitigates her clumsiness at this time of the cycle, and yet another has asked to lead the team fitness sessions because she feels brilliant and wants to share that energy to motivate others. If everyone is tuned in and working with their cycle, the whole squad benefits as a consequence.

How to master your menstrual cycle

- **Track your cycle**
  Data is queen, and the more information you have about your body the better.

- **Be the best version of you on any day of your cycle**
  We're past the stage of leaving success to chance. There's enough knowledge to enable you to make sure you can manage your symptoms well so you can do whatever you need to on any day of the month.

- **Talk openly**
  If it's relevant, talk to others who need to know what's happening with your cycle – it might be a partner, colleague, manager, trainer or physiotherapist. If you think it will help them to understand what your cycle is doing to you, and will help them to help you, talk to them about it.

Chapter 4

Your Body on Birth Control

'Hi, my name is . . .'

Much like Zendaya, Rihanna and Adele, the pill is influential enough to go by a single name. Despite there being hundreds of thousands of other tablets available to us through modern medicine, when you say 'the pill' everyone knows exactly what you're talking about. That's pretty incredible. Since its introduction in 1950, the development of the hormonal contraceptive pill has caused a huge shift in women's ownership of their reproductive rights. Unlike the condom which was largely in the control of men, the pill gave women control over this aspect of their bodies and meant that having sex could be a completely separate endeavour from making babies. The pill's arrival challenged social, political and religious viewpoints about women.

The pill marked the start of an explosion in hormonal contraceptives. Through greater use of the pill, we learned more about the potential side effects of synthetic oestrogens and progestins, and about the doses that were safe, tolerable and effective for women. By the 1990s, new hormone-administering methods were introduced, some offering long-term hormonal delivery, such as the implant and intrauterine devices, in contrast to the daily dose of the pill.

The pill soon became used not just for contraceptive reasons, but to make menstrual cycles more predictable and to alleviate menstrual cycle symptoms or heavy periods that significantly impacted women's lives. It became prescribed to manage other medical conditions, too, such as acne and endometriosis.

While the introduction of hormonal contraception was itself a revolution, we think there needs to be a revolution in how each woman makes the decision to use it, and if so, which type is best for them. As with most prescription medicine, women often find themselves at the mercy of the prescriber – that person's preference, their budget and their experience of what has worked in others; or people glean anecdotal information from their friends about how a certain solution has worked for them. This approach doesn't take into account what effect it might have on *your* body, *your* health and *your* active lifestyle. In trying to find the best type of hormonal contraceptive for an individual, there remains a 'see how you go' approach, where we have to spend up to three months, and sometimes longer, using one type before we can know if it suits us. Some women suffer horrendous side effects before deciding to stick or twist.

It's not just about reproduction

The use of the pill has increased by 35% worldwide over the past twenty-five years, and it's the most common hormonal contraceptive method in Europe, where it's more widely used than across the rest of the world.[1] In the UK, 50% of active women aged eighteen to thirty use hormonal contraception, and for active women in their twenties this can be as high as 66%, dropping to about 11% for those in their mid-forties.

With so many varied experiences of using hormonal contraception existing within the female population, including her own mental health issues that arose through taking the pill, Alice Pelton established The Lowdown,[2] a digital platform where women can review contraceptives and share credible, real-world advice about their options. Being able to find out more about the effects of hormonal contraception is vital when choosing the option that's right for you because the physiological effects of these synthetic hormones don't just influence the reproductive system; they can have consequences throughout the body that influence your health and performance for better or worse. It's astounding how little we know about their effects on our bodies and minds outside their impact on our reproductive system. Over the past few years, a body of evidence has been emerging that shows how they affect the non-reproductive systems in our bodies, and with this evidence comes an opportunity to empower women to make informed decisions about which type of hormonal contraception is right for them in the context of their life, their relationships and their fitness goals.

It's not binary

We often get asked by women whether hormonal contraceptives are 'good' or 'bad' for them, or which pill is 'better'. It's not quite as simple as that. Every woman will have different reasons why they might want or need to take the pill. However, we often see the pill used as a 'quick fix' for more moderate cycle problems, or worse, problems that have a root cause elsewhere, leaving the source of the problem unexplored. Symptoms of other health issues can be masked by the pill and can have long-term health implications if left unresolved.

In a study of Danish athletic women, 60% of hormonal contraceptive users were using it for 'menstrual management' – that is, making their cycle more predictable for the convenience of their active lifestyle.[3] Hormonal contraception is often an excellent strategy to make your body more predictable in terms of menstrual symptoms or bleeding, but moving from having a natural cycle, which can have lots of benefits for your short- and long-term health, to completely suppressing it with the pill, is an extreme move. Most hormonal contraceptives supress your body's own production of cycle hormones by delivering synthetic hormones instead. To take the major step of temporarily removing your natural cycle should involve a full discussion of the pros and cons and knowing the range of hormonal contraceptive options available to you. Yet most women don't embark upon hormonal contraceptive use as fully informed as they could be.

Before we go into the science behind the effects that hormonal contraceptives can have on the body and brain beyond preventing pregnancy, let's have a brief look at the options available and how they work. Having this knowledge puts us in a good starting position to ask for what we think might suit us best.

A winning combination? The combined oral contraceptive pill

To understand how the pill works, we must think back to the menstrual cycle. In the second half of the cycle – the luteal phase, when progesterone is peaking, oestrogen is elevated and ovulation has just taken place – the brain stops sending reproductive signals to the uterus until the next cycle begins. The pill tricks the brain daily into thinking we are in that second half of the menstrual cycle by delivering a synthetic version of oestrogen and progesterone. That way, the brain remains in its 'sitting back and relaxing mode' and doesn't stimulate ovulation because it thinks ovulation has just happened. Preventing ovulation is the primary way the pill prevents pregnancy. No egg released means the sperm has nothing to fertilize, and no baby can be conceived.

The combined oral contraceptive pill (COCP) contains a synthetic version of oestrogen (in the form of ethinyl oestradiol) and of progesterone (progestin), and is delivered in phases: twenty-one days of synthetic hormone delivery and seven days where we either stop taking the pill or the pills in the packet are a placebo. Then the 'pseudo cycle' starts again – 'pseudo cycle' because the pill suppresses our natural menstrual cycle.

We bleed when we're on the pill because during the seven pill-free or placebo-pill days, the synthetic hormone levels drop, triggering what's called a withdrawal bleed. This is normally much lighter than a regular period because the lining of the uterus hasn't been built up as it would have been in a natural cycle. Having a withdrawal bleed is certainly not a medical necessity; it's actually just a relic from when the pill was developed in the 1960s, when it was thought that women would be reassured by their pill cycle mimicking a natural menstrual cycle. Plus, it was culturally more acceptable for women to still have a monthly bleed. It's now established that because the lining of the uterus is kept relatively thin and healthy when using hormonal contraceptives, there's no physiological or medical reason to have a bleed or a break in your pills, and new guidelines in 2019 from the Faculty of Sexual and Reproductive Healthcare's Clinical Effectiveness Unit at the Royal College of Obstetricians and Gynaecologists say that it's perfectly safe not to take a break between pill packs.[4] These guidelines apply to the monophasic COCP which deliver the same level of hormone per pill throughout the pack. This means a woman can choose whether she wants to have a regular bleed or not; many decide to take the packets back-to-back with no withdrawal bleeds.

POP the progestogen–only pill

The progestogen-only pill (POP), as its name suggests, contains only progestin – synthetic progestogen. It works in much the same way as the COCP because the high level of progestin in the pill tricks your brain into thinking you're in the luteal phase of your menstrual cycle all the time. As with the COCP, you don't ovulate because your body thinks it has already done that. You take one pill a day for twenty-eight days and move straight on to the next packet without a break. About 50% of women find that they don't bleed at all on this type of contraception, and others have very light 'breakthrough' bleeding caused by the shedding of a small amount of the uterus lining that is being kept fairly thin by taking the pill. The old-generation POP, known as the mini pill, has a strict criterion that requires it to be taken within the same three-hour time slot daily to be effective. The new-generation pills have a twelve-hour window within which you can safely take the pill and retain the benefits.

Powerful progestins – and how they might affect your strength and power

Although most combined pills use the same type of synthetic oestrogen, the progestin in COCPs and POPs can vary. The different types have been grouped into four so-called 'generations', based on what they're made from and when they first became available. It's important to know what type of progestin is being used in your pill because different generations can have different side effects. Knowing what the pill contains can help you spot any potential issues before deciding whether it's right for you, or troubleshoot any problems that crop up once you start taking it.

Most progestins are derived not from progesterone, but from testosterone. This means that they can sometimes have what we call an androgenic action on your body – in other words, they act on your body the same way androgen hormones, such as testosterone, would do. This can manifest itself through acne, weight gain and increased body hair in unwelcome places. First- and second-generation progestins have the most testosterone-like side effects, whereas third-generation progestins do less of the masculinizing, and many women on this type notice no unwanted side effects. Fourth-generation progestins are slightly different in that they are anti-androgenic, meaning they act in the opposite way of their masculinizing predecessors; their chemical make-up blocks the effects of testosterone on the body. The pill with fourth-generation progestins is often used to treat severe acne or hirsutism, the medical term for abnormal growth of hair on a woman's face or body. The trade-off for this effective treatment is that they have also been found to significantly lower women's libido.[5]

Long-Acting Reversible Contraceptives (LARCs)

LARCs are forms of progestin-only hormonal contraceptive device that have long-lasting effects over a long period of time after implantation or insertion. Their influence is reversible because, even though you can have them inside your body for a long time, as soon as you have them removed (and you can at any time), the effects of their synthetic hormones soon wear off.

The implant

The implant is a small, non-biodegradable rod, about the size of a matchstick, that contains progestin. Fitting it requires a minor surgical procedure, with a small injection of local anaesthetic, in which the implant is inserted under the skin on the inside of a woman's non-dominant upper arm. The implant is what Dr Bella likes to call a 'fit and forget' type of hormonal contraception: provided you don't have unwanted side effects, once it's fitted, you're covered for – and can forget about – both contraception and cycle-symptom management for up to three years.

When the implant is first inserted, there can be a light bleed, and in some women this can last for up to three months. While for 25% of women this prolonged bleeding leads them to have the implant removed, for most the bleeding will taper off, and 20% of women end up having no further bleeding for the life of the implant.[6] It's important to remember that although this is a long-acting hormonal contraception, you can ask for it to be removed at any time, so you don't have to wait the full three years while it's effective if you're not tolerating it or no longer want it.

The intrauterine system (IUS)

Another 'fit and forget' type of hormonal contraception is the intrauterine system, often called the coil. Not to be confused with the copper coil (which is a non-hormonal coil), this coil is a T-shaped plastic device that is inserted into the uterus and releases a very small amount of progestin directly on to the lining of the uterus at a low, steady rate. Unlike the pill, the coil does not work by preventing ovulation. Instead, it keeps the lining of the uterus thin – though still healthy – so that any fertilized egg would not be able to implant there and develop into a pregnancy. It also thickens the cervical fluid so sperm can't get in there in the first place.

The coil gets to work as soon as it's fitted, releasing its progestin in the uterus and encouraging any lining that's already there to shed, to get it down to the thin layer that prevents pregnancy. This means that many women experience some period-like bleeding when they first have the coil inserted.

Due to the uterine lining being kept thin, many women find that their periods significantly lighten, or even stop, when they have the IUS fitted. This is why an IUS is often offered to women who have heavy periods. Once in place, an IUS is effective for five years.

The main difference between an IUS and other implants or the pill is that because an IUS delivers a small dose of progestin straight to the uterus, the progestin doesn't travel around your body and therefore has fewer effects on your natural hormonal responses. This means that about a year after inserting the IUS, the brain can start to send its normal signals to the ovaries, and a natural rhythm of hormone release across the menstrual cycle might resume, albeit without a period, because the IUS keeps the uterus lining thin. In one study of women who were fitted with an IUS, after one year following insertion 45% of cycles were ovulatory (in other words, the cycle hormones are all doing their thing), and in another study, four years after insertion 75% of cycles were ovulatory.[7]

It's easy for your doctor to remove your IUS and, if required, insert a new one, either at the end of its five-year lifespan or sooner, if that's what you decide.

We think the IUS offers an amazing combination of contraceptive protection – it's one of the most effective forms of contraception available – and symptom management, together with the benefits of retaining a natural cycle and reaping the hormonal rewards of your natural monthly oestrogen and progesterone peaks. Unfortunately, the insertion process often puts women off having it in the first place. Some women find it very painful or uncomfortable, especially if they have not had children. The coil is pushed through the hole in your cervix, which can often give an intense, period-like pain that can last about ten seconds, though some women suffer pain or cramping for a few hours after insertion. If you were to talk to ten women who have had the coil inserted, you would hear ten different experiences – from not really being bothered by insertion, all the way to nearly passing out because of the pain. Also, there are different brands of IUS available for women with a smaller or tighter cervix that can be easier to insert.

The media coverage of women experiencing severe or unbearable pain during a coil insertion has led to important reviews and discussions of how this procedure is performed. The bottom line is that no woman should ever endure severe or unbearable pain when having the IUS fitted (or during any medical procedure) and this issue should be discussed and planned well in advance of it being inserted. The majority of women Dr Bella sees tolerate the insertion very well and do not need additional pain relief. This includes taking NSAIDs (like ibuprofen) thirty minutes prior to the procedure, using a lidocaine gel or spray to coat the cervix during insertion, or, in some cases, a local anaesthetic injection directly into the cervix to numb it completely. Most coils can be inserted at your doctor's surgery or local sexual health clinic, but if necessary, you can be seen in your local hospital, with insertion under sedation or a general anaesthetic. The most important message is that women should not silently endure a painful procedure and should speak up if in pain. So, don't let insertion be the thing that stops you using the coil, if in all other ways it's a great solution for you. Talk to your doctor or sexual health nurse about your anxieties and see whether it can be fitted in a way that feels right for you and your concerns.

The contraceptive injection

There are two types of contraceptive injections available in the UK at the time of writing. Each contains progestin and is given every ten to twelve weeks. The main difference between the two is that one is self-administered, whereas the other must be given by a doctor or nurse, meaning you have to regularly visit your health centre. The benefits of the injection are, like the implant and IUS, that they last a long time and are very effective. The injection is not reversible, however, so once you've had it, you can't simply 'take it out' if it doesn't suit you.

When Emma was working in Olympic and Paralympic sport, there was a reluctance to give female athletes contraceptive injections due to research showing that it affects bone-mineral density, heightening the risk of bone fractures.[8] Furthermore, this effect increased with longer-term use and may not be completely reversible. This is concerning for younger women because we lay down all our bone density in the years until we are thirty, and from then on, unfortunately, it declines with age. Good diet and exercise can slow down this decline, but a really important factor is to make sure you have as high a peak in bone density as you can by the time you are thirty. If you impair the process before this, through something like the contraceptive injection (or by losing your periods, known as amenorrhea), then you reduce your chances of a high peak bone mass. For older women, maintaining bone mass is a priority for health and well-being and so again, a risk of losing bone density through use of the injection is a consideration. Because of this, there are strong warnings on the injection packaging cautioning that it shouldn't be used for longer than two years, and that using these products might increase the risk of osteoporosis and bone fractures later in life.

Myth busting

Women's health is no stranger to myths, and when it comes to hormonal contraception there are some specific ones we'd love to bust.

Myth: You still get periods when you're on the pill

On some pills, women have a monthly bleed but because the pill suppresses our natural menstrual cycle, this bleed is not a period, it is a withdrawal bleed – it is the body's response to a withdrawal from the pill's artificial hormones on pill-free days of your pill cycle or on the days when the pill you take doesn't contain any synthetic hormones. This bleed isn't part of a menstrual cycle like your period; it's part of a pill cycle. It's important for active women to understand that having a regular withdrawal bleed when you are using hormonal contraception isn't the same as having a regular period. In women not using hormonal contraception, the regular and smooth arrival of their period each month is an indicator that they are in good overall health with a well-balanced diet that meets the energy demands of their lives and exercise schedule. Women on the pill cannot use their withdrawal bleed to indicate this kind of energy balance or sign of overall good health; they need to find other ways to be diligent about making sure they fuel their training well and don't ignore health issues that don't feel right to them.

Myth: Hormonal contraception eliminates all cycle symptoms

Often women find that using hormonal contraception gets rid of some pretty unpleasant menstrual cycle symptoms. In fact, over half of women using the pill do so, at least in part, specifically to lessen cycle symptoms.[9] But for some women, contrary to removing unwanted symptoms associated with the menstrual cycle, hormonal contraception can bring them on, including continuous bleeding, headaches, acne, moodiness, reduced motivation, a 'flat line' feeling and weight gain.[10]

For women who go on hormonal contraception to alleviate certain cycle symptoms, it can be really disheartening to find that a new set of equally uncomfortable and painful symptoms appear when they start taking the pill. It's important not to think that this means the pill isn't for you, because, as we've seen, there are many types of pill and they can each have very different effects on individuals. We've seen lots of women abandon the use of hormonal contraception after their first try or continue using it even though it's not right for them, because they don't feel confident asking for an alternative. So, don't be afraid to go back to your doctor and ask for a solution that works for you.

One last point: because of possible side effects and symptoms, we discourage women from starting on a new hormonal contraception close to a big event if there's no urgency for contraceptive purposes. Whether it's the London Marathon, a sponsored swim you're doing to raise money for charity, or you're starting a new job, plan the timing as kindly and usefully as possible for yourself and your goals.

Myth: Hormonal contraception can be used to kick-start your cycle

There's a lot of bad practice when it comes to prescribing the pill to improve menstrual health. Hormonal contraceptives suppress the menstrual cycle, and because of that, they can't be used to kick-start the cycle in girls where periods haven't yet begun, or in women whose periods have disappeared, or to 'repair' a very irregular cycle. The problem with starting hormonal contraception when you haven't been having periods, or when you have very irregular periods, is that the pseudo-cycle brought on by the hormonal contraception can mask what is fundamentally wrong with your menstrual cycle. It might be due to an energy imbalance preventing ovulation, or to polycystic ovaries or chronic stress, but the key here is to use the menstrual cycle dysfunction as your cue to get to the root cause. If you do that when your body first starts signalling to you, then the strategies for regaining a healthy menstrual cycle and not suffering more widespread consequences may turn out to be quite simple. Your body will give you the thumbs-up that your strategies are working, because you'll see an improvement in your menstrual health, whether that be more regular periods or a reappearance of periods after their absence. Hormonal contraception masks the problem, and it masks your ability to see if things are improving because you've taken away this 'vital sign'. In short, using hormonal contraception is not a good idea if you haven't found or addressed the root cause of primary or secondary amenorrhoea, which means, respectively, not starting, or starting and then later on losing, your periods.

Myth: There's no point cycle tracking when you use hormonal contraceptives

Even though you're not having a menstrual cycle when you're using hormonal contraceptives, it's a good idea to track your mood, energy levels, appetite, libido, motivation to train, performance and anything else that is meaningful for you as you start taking hormonal contraception or change to a new type. Just like tracking your menstrual cycle, this insight will help you decide if you've found what's right for you and will also give you lots of information to share with your doctor if you haven't.

Myth: It takes time to get pregnant after using hormonal contraception

If you are sexually active and you stop using hormonal contraception because it isn't right for you, it's important to remember that you need to use another form of contraception as soon as you stop. For contraception such as the coil, where ovulation is still occurring when the coil is in place, once the coil is removed, fertility should quickly return to normal. This means you can get pregnant as soon as you have had your coil removed. For other methods, there is a variable time frame within which women return to having an ovulatory cycle. It could happen straight away, it could take a few months, either is within the bounds of normal and healthy.

Side effects that might sideline you

As an active woman, your choice of hormonal contraceptive should also take into account how the side effects of certain contraceptives might impact your enjoyment or performance in the particular types of sport, exercise or other physical activity you like to do. Will it give you symptoms that interfere with your motivation to train or your ability to build strength, for example? Questions like these can become part of your discussion with your doctor – let them know that your sport or being active is important to you and that you would like a contraceptive that doesn't compromise your ability to train and perform to the best of your ability.

We often hear from women who have been on the pill for a long time and only realize how much it's been affecting them when they stop taking it. Take the swimmer who described not being able to experience the emotional highs and lows associated with competing – the anxiety when standing on the starting blocks and the elation that came from winning a race were all slightly numbed; the rower who told us that while she was on the pill her mood was permanently lower than she felt it should be – when she came off it, her instincts were proven right and her mood returned to normal, to her great relief; the CrossFitter who found her muscle mass and strength diminished when she went on the pill. These women's experiences made us want to look deeper into the science of hormonal contraception and its potential impact on exercise and sports performance.

Our investigation turned up some interesting emerging findings about the influence of hormonal contraception on active women's health and well-being. We need to emphasize the word 'emerging' here – if you think back to how few women have been studied in sports science research to date, that's nothing compared to how little evidence we have about what synthetic hormones in contraception might be doing in active women's bodies. But we certainly have enough to pique our curiosity, especially when the science matches up with the experiences that active women share with us so often. The next sections take a deeper dive into some of the side effects which might sideline us.

Taking the pill can be super-stressful

A study of over two hundred women suggests that taking the pill can cause high levels of stress hormones to continually circulate in a woman's body (for as long as she's on the pill).[11] This is bad news; the effects of chronic stress on our overall health is well-documented – it's not good for us. Chronic stress can lead to chronic inflammation, which has been shown to affect our immune function, cardiovascular health and cognitive function, and to increase the risk of depression.[12] These findings are confirmed by a study on women preparing for the Rio Olympic Games in which the stress and inflammation markers of a group of athletes taking the oral contraceptive pill were compared with a group of athletes having a natural cycle.[13] The study found that 36% of athletes on the pill had markers of systemic inflammation that were three times higher than the levels found in the non-pill takers. Although elevated levels of markers of stress and inflammation are a normal part of the exercise-recovery-adaptation process in humans, particularly athletes, the fact that sportswomen taking the pill have significantly higher markers than their peers not on the pill is currently being investigated by researchers to examine the effect on their performance, ability to recover and adapt, and their long-term health.

One of the first times we heard about the pill having a potentially negative effect on performance was in a case study presented in 2017 on an athlete who was underperforming and not adapting to training as expected, with no obvious reason why.[14] In sport we call this UPS: unexplained underperformance syndrome – when an athlete doesn't get fitter, stronger or more powerful even when they are training hard to make progress. When the athlete took a blood test, she showed elevated markers of oxidative stress and higher levels of circulating cortisol, which you might see in someone with chronic stress and which are certainly not optimal for an athlete. One of the strategies to help this athlete recover was to take her off the pill, based on what we know about its ability to impact our baseline levels of stress hormones. Soon afterwards, her blood profile had returned to normal and she no longer suffered from chronic stress. Coming off the pill, along with addressing some nutritional factors and improving the quality of her recovery, was part of this athlete's strategy to return to peak performance. It's hard to know whether, among the other things she did, coming off the pill made the defining difference, but it's acknowledged that it was an important factor in her recovery.

Don't take the highs with the lows

In the face of threat or stress, our sympathetic nervous system kicks in: our adrenal glands release adrenaline – the surge you feel – making your heart race, your breathing speed up and your pupils dilate; then cortisol rises, which increases sugars in your blood, giving you immediate energy. This combination is our body's natural fight-or-flight response. You don't necessarily feel the cortisol in the way that you do the adrenaline, but it plays a big part in managing the stress response you're having by redistributing energy to body parts that need a boost, like your muscles. Cortisol also promotes perceptual vigilance, learning and memory. This means that it allows us to remember and etch into our brains whatever was causing the stress, so later down the line we don't find it quite as alarming or stressful. It helps us adapt to be more resilient in the future.

Interestingly, although there is evidence that women on the pill have elevated levels of baseline cortisol, they consistently show a blunted, or in some cases, absent cortisol response to stress. The adrenaline rush happens, and they 'feel' stressed, but the cortisol peak doesn't happen, so they don't manage the stress, learn from it or adapt to it.[15] In one study, women performed an exercise test, cycling to exhaustion.[16] Half of these exercisers were on the pill, the other half were not. During the cycling, the physiological responses of both groups of women were the same, and after the exercise, as expected, mood was improved in all women (exercise is awesome like that). However, in women on the pill, the cortisol response at the end of the exercise was significantly lower than in those who were not; their stress response was blunted. This is important for active women because our body's response to exercise, including the cortisol rise, is what it needs to recover from that exercise and adapt to it, staying healthy and growing fitter and stronger in the process.[17]

Making muscle

The pill can also influence our ability to gain strength and muscle mass, as experienced by the CrossFitter mentioned earlier. This might be because taking the pill can influence another group of hormones in our body: androgens. Androgens are hormones that influence growth, including growth of muscle, in both men and women. We often think of androgens as male hormones, and they are produced in much higher quantities in males, but women produce small amounts of these hormones naturally, too, and one of their jobs is to help us repair and grow muscle in response to exercise. One of the main androgen hormones is testosterone, from which progestin, present in the pill to varying degrees, is derived. The types of contraceptive pill that are used to treat symptoms such as acne and body hair are anti-androgenic, meaning they suppress the effect of our natural testosterone thereby limiting the body's ability to build muscle after exercise.

One study has found that women not taking the pill, and who have a healthy menstrual cycle, gained significantly more muscle mass than women on the pill, following a ten-week resistance-training programme.[18] Women not on the pill had about a 3.5% increase in muscle mass after this training, compared with a 2.5% increase in women using the pill. But the most interesting finding came when the researchers zoomed in on the group taking the pill. They compared women in that group according to whether they used the anti-androgenic pill or a different type and saw no increase in strength after the ten-week regime in those using anti-androgenic pills compared with a 2.5 % increase in the women who used other pills. It's not straightforward, and there's still much research to do into this phenomenon, but it's possible that strength gain may be affected by the type of pill a woman is taking.

Bodyweight battles

We know that bodyweight can fluctuate across the menstrual cycle, but it can also be affected by hormonal contraception too. Research shows that while the pill might not directly cause weight gain, it might affect behaviours that can cause women to gain weight when they start taking the pill.[19] It's thought that the synthetic hormones might increase appetite, decrease feelings of being full, and increase visceral (tummy) fat deposits. The way fat is distributed across our bodies is largely influenced by hormones – it's why, when we go through puberty as girls, our body shape starts changing and we deposit fat on our bums, hips and breasts. Men tend to deposit fat around their tummy, so women who find that this starts happening to them when they start using the pill may be experiencing one of those masculinizing effects of the progestins in the pill.

Your mental health and birth control

There are some important and interesting findings emerging that detail how our brain is influenced by hormonal contraceptives. Evidence shows that, in women on the pill, there are structural and functional changes to the brain, particularly in the hippocampus, the part of our brain that helps us learn and remember. Women on the pill have been shown to give up more quickly on unsolvable word puzzles and perform worse in difficult tests, compared with women not on the pill.[20] We've spoken to active women who've described a slowness in their decision-making or ability to read the game when on the pill, and while there isn't yet any specific sports research on this topic, there's certainly some correlation between the stories we hear from women and what the science currently shows.

There's also compelling evidence for the link between the use of hormonal contraception and poor mental health.[21] Denmark leads in this field of research as it keeps nationwide registers of all its citizens on a number of health and social issues. It can therefore conduct nationwide surveys, resulting in valuable analysis on the connections between people's social behaviour and their health outcomes. It's from these registers that we learn a lot about the links between taking the pill and mental health disorders.

A Danish nationwide study has found that women who are on hormonal contraceptives are 50% more likely to be diagnosed with depression within six months of starting to use it, and 40% more likely to be prescribed antidepressants than women with a natural cycle. The data from this study also shows that, in younger women, aged fifteen to nineteen, the depression risk is even greater. This is extraordinary and makes us wonder why we don't talk about this risk more openly, or why doctors don't at the very least make women aware of it when we hand over the pill.

In the previous chapter we discussed the calming effects that progesterone can have on the brain. There is growing research that shows that the pill works in the same circuits of the brain but in the opposite way, making people feel anxious, overwhelmed and depressed. Research also shows that women on the pill are more likely to have a blunted emotional response to happy things and not to experience activity in the reward centres of the brain in the same way as those who aren't on the pill.[22]

A fall in fitness

While your athletic performance capacities, such as strength, speed and aerobic fitness, are not affected by your menstrual cycle, scientists are unsure whether the same can be said for hormonal contraception. A review of all studies of fitness markers in hormonal contraception users versus those with a natural menstrual cycle found 'a potentially negative influence' on performance when using an oral contraceptive pill.[23] A few of these studies were highlighted as having strong research design, i.e. the results were objective, reliable and valid. These possibly stood out because 64% of the research was considered moderate- or low-quality when it comes to researching the menstrual cycle and performance. It's disappointing to see such a large proportion of research being conducted on active women that is not considered robust enough for the outcomes to be trusted. However, a strong research design was used in a study from the University of California that tested the effects of the pill on women's aerobic capacity, a marker of endurance fitness.[24] Women were tested throughout their natural menstrual cycle, and then all participants took the same pill for four months. This meant that all women acted as their own control group: each woman was in both the menstrual cycle group and the pill group. While aerobic capacity remained stable across the natural menstrual cycle, as we've seen in numerous other studies, when the women started taking the pill, aerobic fitness decreased by 11% and their peak power on a cycling test decreased by 8%.

In another study, this time in Canada, aerobic capacity was measured in active women across their natural menstrual cycle and then participants were assigned to take either a hormonal contraceptive pill or a placebo pill.[25] This research found that when women were using the pill, they had a 4.7% decline in their aerobic capacity compared with a 1.5% improvement in the placebo group. Those on the pill also showed an increase in body fat.

This data is fascinating because it suggests that in some women there are quantifiable effects on their bodies resulting from taking the pill, beyond contraception. We eagerly await more research into other forms of hormonal contraceptive so that we can fully understand the impact of all forms of hormonal contraceptive on the female body.

Emma

When I show athletes research about how hormonal contraception might influence a woman's physiology and neurobiology, they start asking how they will know if their pill (which they have often been on for years) is affecting them in this way, and, as a competitive athlete, whether they should stop using it? My answer is always, if you are thriving on this pill – that is, you are fit and healthy, you are adapting to your training, performing well and you feel good – then there is no reason to change anything. You've probably found a great solution in what you are currently using. The only way to find out if your performance is compromised would be to come off the pill and track changes over a few months, including your results in fitness tests and in training. That's your choice, and you now make it from a more informed position.

Your body, your choice

Not all women will experience these performance-impacting effects when taking hormonal contraception. Some of you will have been happily using hormonal contraceptives for years, if not decades, and you may feel that none of this applies. But some of you may be starting to realize why you feel like you do and can now put your finger on something that you weren't able to previously.

Whatever the case, we know that you are now much better informed about what hormonal contraception is and what effect it might have on you as an active woman. Now you have the power to choose what you do next!

For us, it's about weighing up all this information, along with your reasons for wanting to use hormonal contraception, in the context of your life, your sport, your health and your relationships, and making an informed choice. One thing's for sure: this broader view and emerging evidence hasn't been presented in the context of sport and exercise until now. It isn't meant to take away from the fact that there's lots of evidence to show that the pill is effective as birth control, and for women with certain hormonally triggered mood disorders, endometriosis, acne and severe period pain. But when that pill is prescribed to you by your health professional, make sure that it is accompanied by the information you need to help you make an informed decision about which pill might be right for you. Arm yourself with the full facts about the positive and negative effects each solution might have and give yourself time to try different hormonal contraceptive solutions until you find the perfect fit.

How to crack contraception

- **What's the problem?**
  Have a big think about the problem you're trying to
  solve by using hormonal contraception. Is it to avoid an

unplanned pregnancy or cycle symptoms, or because periods are an inconvenience? Is it because your cycle isn't working well, or at all? Once you know why you want or need to use hormonal contraception, you can start to make an informed choice about what might work best for you.

- **What are you afraid of?**
  If you love the idea of the coil but are worried about insertion, make sure you explore the options of how to remove that anxiety or pain as a barrier for using the type of hormonal contraception you want to.

- **If it ain't broke, don't fix it**
  If whatever you're taking is working for you, carry on. Hormonal contraception by design is great, we just need to be as educated as we can be about it.

- **Take a holistic approach**
  Be holistic in your approach to solving the problem: hormonal contraception may turn out to be the best solution, but there may be other options out there that could help.

- **Know yourself**
  Be aware of how healthy you are. If you're on hormonal contraception, you won't be getting the monthly signal, each time your period arrives, that your body is healthy. So be vigilant about things like the balance between how much energy you're expending and how much you are taking in, how well you recover from training or how you're managing stress.

Chapter 5

Perfecting Your Pelvic Floor

A solid foundation: your pelvic floor

For those of you who think knowing about the pelvic floor is a mum thing, think again. Why do all women need to know about the pelvic floor? Because you've all got one. In fact, everybody has a pelvic floor and you can't replace it, unlike your teeth (which you take impeccable daily care of, right?). A quarter of all women aged twenty or above report at least one symptom of pelvic floor dysfunction like leaking urine.[1] Pelvic floor dysfunction is neither exclusively a mum thing or an old woman thing; it's an everywoman thing. If you manage to remain symptom free in your twenties and thirties, fast-forward, just for an instant, a couple of decades, at which point – trust us – you could be wishing you'd paid more attention to your pelvic floor. Like so many parts of our bodies, it will stop working as well as you age, regardless of how physically fit you are right now, whether you birthed kids or intend to have them, whether you are currently experiencing issues with your pelvic floor or not.

Along with so much of what's in this book, it's unlikely that anyone has ever told you what we are about to share, yet it will transform your lifestyle and well-being. While the pelvic floor is rarely on the radar of young, fit, active women, we at The Well HQ feel strongly that it should be, as we know that leaking urine (or the fear of leaking urine) leads to anxiety and loss of self-confidence, and stops many women exercising or playing the sport they love. We encourage you to bring it into conversations with other women you know and those who support you with your health, from doctors and nurses to trainers and coaches.

As with so many important body systems, we don't notice a healthy pelvic floor until it goes wrong. You don't appreciate how well it's doing its job any more than you celebrate your digestive tract after you've eaten a meal and effortlessly processed it or congratulate your lungs for keeping up with your pace as you pound through intervals in a spin class. But when your pelvic floor isn't working as it should, it can be anything from a distraction to a lifestyle encumbrance. The first sign of an unhealthy pelvic floor is often leaking urine, which catches you unaware but will quickly become a persistent reminder that all is not well. Many women resort to wearing pads, and some have reported they go as far as to alter their drinking behaviour so that they don't have to use the toilet, both of which impact our health and well-being, and are merely a sticking plaster on a more deep-rooted issue.

In an open letter to *Canadian Running* magazine in 2019, women's health physio Julie Wiebe explained the relevance of a dysfunctional pelvic floor, writing that leaking is a sign your body isn't working well and if you swapped out the word 'leaking' for the word 'pain' there would be much more attention paid to pelvic floor dysfunction.[2] Most of us, certainly athletes and coaches, don't tolerate pain – it's interpreted as a clear signal that help is needed. A sub-optimal pelvic floor should also be a signal to get some help and look at the big picture, not just to manage the symptoms but to piece together other issues we're experiencing in terms of breathing dynamics, bladder and bowel issues, or hip or lower back pain, any of which may correlate with leaking.

Evidence has been emerging over the past few years about the prevalence of pelvic floor dysfunction in active women, with rates ranging from 8% to 80%, depending on the training volumes and impact levels of the sport.[3] We know that female athletes have much higher rates of urinary incontinence. Annoyingly, though, not enough is known about why. So, when Baz and Emma toured the UK giving education sessions for support teams, coaches and athletes in Olympic and Paralympic programmes, we expected this to come up as a common issue. Yet no one brought it up at all. And when we asked if leaking was common among female athletes, the sports doctors told us no athletes were presenting with this problem. But when we asked the coaches, they said, 'Oh yes, all the athletes wet themselves,' and the athletes responded with, 'We thought that was a normal part of training hard.'

This example demonstrates beautifully (or frustratingly!) how pelvic floor dysfunction has become totally normalized and underreported within exercise and sport. Very few perceive this common condition as a problem or a performance issue, as they should, and as a result it goes untreated. The situation reflects attitudes in our wider society, where there is also little concern about it. This needs to change.

What is the pelvic floor, anyway?

When Baz decided to become a women's health coach, she was embarrassed to admit that she didn't know what the pelvic floor was – she was thirty-eight years old, had been an elite athlete, birthed two babies, and had never known what the pelvic floor was, nor what it did. She vaguely knew it was around the bottom area, as most of us do, but that was it. So, although this next bit may seem a bit boring, it's essential knowledge – for all of us.

The pelvic floor is a group of muscles and connective tissue that attach within your pelvis, suspended like a hammock, connecting your pubic bone at the front to your coccyx at the back. This is as much as we need to know – women's health physios and gynaecologists need to know plenty more about the anatomy of the pelvic floor, but for everyone else that's enough.

Anatomy of the pelvic floor

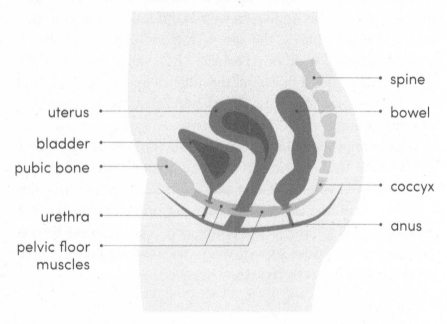

Anatomy of the pelvic floor

Like every muscle, the pelvic floor should be able to contract and relax, and it should have a good range of motion. This is a key point because mostly women believe that if they have an issue with it, they must do more pelvic floor exercises, but that's an oversimplification. Like any part of the body that's not working as it should, the fix is rarely off the shelf or standardized.

The pelvic floor should be able to:

- **Keep you dry**
  Your pelvic floor should be able to stop you from leaking urine, wind or stools. Which means that if you are doing impact sports, such as netball, sprinting or trampolining, your pelvic floor needs to be much stronger than it does for someone who goes to the gym every so often or whose exercise choice is walking.

- **Relax when necessary**
  Your pelvic floor should be able to relax enough when you're on the toilet that you can fully empty your bladder and bowel. Research has shown that the women who are unable to relax their pelvic floor completely often suffer with bloating, constipation, sexual pain and lower back pain as a result of not being able to empty their bowels completely when they go to the toilet.[4]

The pelvic floor is part of your core, which also comprises your back, abs and diaphragm, and must be as strong, mobile and coordinated as the rest of the unit. It rises and falls with your breathing. It should also be strong enough to keep you dry when the body is doing more (e.g. running, lifting weights, jumping on a trampoline), which is why the more exercise you do, the more conditioned your pelvic floor needs to be.

It's important to note that the pelvic floor is not designed to be clenched for ages. You can't go for a run and hold your pelvic floor throughout. You can't do a vinyasa flow sequence and keep your pelvic floor lifted. It's designed to move with your breath and resist pressure from above (e.g. from laughing, coughing, sneezing, holding your breath) and from below (such as from running or jumping).

Taking back control: how to do a pelvic floor exercise

Women are generally sold a lie about how easy it is to do their pelvic floor exercises, but you can't squeeze your vagina at the traffic lights with a car full of kids! As Baz knows from when she's coaching a room full of women to do this, the level of concentration when you're first mastering your pelvic floor exercises is significant. You need to connect with a private, vulnerable and intimate part of yourself (which may trigger some women if they've had a medical or sexual experience that was traumatic). Women therefore need time, safety and practice to master this skill. After a few weeks, it will become a lot easier and you can do it while you wait for the kettle to boil or while brushing your teeth, but in the early days it's really worth giving yourself the time and space to learn how to isolate this part of your body.

Unlike your biceps, you can't see your pelvic floor, so it's hard for most women to work out how to do their exercises. So here are three great visualizations for you, to help identify the area you're working with – give them all a try and see which one works best. Attempt them on your own, in a room with the door shut, so you feel safe, unobserved and relaxed.

Basic pelvic floor exercises

To begin with, try the following in either a seated or lying-down position:

1. Imagine you're picking up a magic bean with your anus and another one with your vagina, in one action, and then let the beans go. Once this feels right, pick up both magic beans again, but this time continue to

draw up your vagina towards your belly button for a couple of seconds; then drop, relax and let go.

2. Imagine you're walking into the ocean. As you go in, you notice tickly little fish starting to nibble at your vulva and anus, and you lift both your vulva and anus away from the fish. Once the fish have swum away, you can relax and let go.

3. Imagine your pelvic floor is a grabber on a toy truck. To begin with, the grabber is open (you're relaxed). Start to close the grabber by drawing the back and front of your pelvic floor together (your coccyx and your pubic-bone area) as if the grabber is pulling up a tampon into your vagina. Then open the grabber to let go.

Once you've worked out which of these visualizations works best for you, aim to do ten lifts and relaxes each day. After you've mastered your exercise while lying down or sitting, progress to doing it while standing. This is key: none of us needs a strong pelvic floor when we're lying down. It's a great place to start, but we need our pelvic floor to work for us when we're standing and moving about.

Advanced pelvic floor exercises

Once you've nailed the basics, we strongly recommend that you add in breathing to your exercise by following this sequence:

1. Inhale softly.
2. Start to exhale slowly and begin your pelvic floor exercise, lifting the vagina and anus up for the length

of the exhale (this takes coordination, as we are often used to relaxing on an exhale, but with pelvic floor exercises we need to draw up the pelvic floor muscle during the exhale).

3. Then relax the pelvic floor as you inhale.
4. Take a moment, and then repeat.

Don't worry if this feels odd – it takes coordination and concentration when you first try to bring your breathing dynamics into your pelvic floor work.

Getting the pelvic floor on to the gym floor

Once you've got the hang of them, you can do your pelvic floor exercises almost anywhere, but you also need to make sure you're protecting and supporting your pelvic floor function when you work out. When it comes to weight training, most coaches teach you to hold your breath – take a deep breath in at the top of your squat, hold it, push the air down, do your lift and as you stand up, start to exhale. We're taught to create as much core tension as possible to allow us to transfer maximum loads through our bodies. The breath-holding technique is an amazing way of creating tone and tension in your core and protecting your back when lifting heavy weights. The only issue with this – and it's a pretty big one – is that women have a vagina! Unlike the other holes in our pelvis, vaginas don't have a sphincter (which keeps our anus and urethra shut until we consciously want to go to the toilet). So, when there's an increase in pressure above the vagina (intra-abdominal pressure, such as when we are holding our breath and lifting a heavy load), our pelvic organs are not supported as well and there is a risk of prolapse, a common pelvic floor issue that can be made worse by breath-holding. If we're doing this breath-hold in every lift, multiple times a week, it can become a problem.

The point is that if you're lifting a middle-weight kettlebell or deadlifting a weight that is reasonable to you, you don't need to hold your breath. The best way to support your pelvic organs is to save the breath-holding until you actually need to be doing it. Strength-and-conditioning coaches, and personal trainers, are increasingly interested in how to support their clients and athletes to train using the female filter by keeping women's bodies in mind, and there are many ways that the pelvic floor can be integrated into gym programming.

Bear in mind that there are a whole host of reasons you may be experiencing pelvic floor issues and that there are different solutions to each problem. Your pelvic floor could be too weak or not coordinated with your core or it could be too tight – also called a hypertonic or non-relaxing pelvic floor, which is more common in active women.[5] In short, there's more to understanding and training your pelvic floor than simply doing pelvic floor exercises, but a good place to start is always by doing some basic pelvic floor exercises, and, if they don't work, finding a women's health physiotherapist.

FAQs

I can feel my tummy/glutes contracting when I do my pelvic floor exercises. Is that OK?

This is very normal but ideally you should work specifically on just the pelvic floor. Try focusing on your pelvic floor without squeezing anything else.

I can only lift for a couple of seconds – is that enough?

Great that you can feel the lift. A couple of seconds is fine but over two to six weeks you should aim to progress towards ten seconds of holding in a standing position.

Why does it feel weird lifting the pelvic floor on the exhale?

Many of us who have done any form of sport, dance or Pilates may have been told to breathe differently, but this is how the pelvic floor works – with the diaphragm. The diaphragm lifts up on the exhale, and so does the pelvic floor. Stick with it: it will come.

Why are these exercises not working for my pelvic floor issues?

Visit your doctor or women's health physiotherapist and tell them what you've been doing, so that they're aware that you're exercising your pelvic floor, but it's not helping. A women's health physio will be able to check whether you're doing your exercise properly, look for underlying causes of dysfunction and come up with a rehabilitation plan that works for you.

Why can't I feel my pelvic floor relaxing?

This is very common. Many of us hold our stomachs in as a habit, and if we're worried about leaking or are feeling anxious generally, we transfer this tension to our pelvic floors. Baz has worked with many women who need to focus purely on the relaxing and letting go, as opposed to the lift. The key to this is to be patient and consistent, and to give yourself time and space to feel the release. One way of doing this is in the bath or shower:

relax and insert your finger into your vagina, feel the muscles then notice what happens when you push down a little bit – you'll quickly feel how high your muscles normally sit and learn what it feels like when they are relaxed.

Why are these exercises so boring?

Yes, they might be boring, but so is cleaning your teeth or washing your face. Baz has worked with many women who hate doing their exercises, are resentful that they have to do them and are really angry that they have to fix what they feel is not their fault. With this mindset it's a battle. Try to see your pelvic floor exercises as a time for you, a time to connect with your body and a sign that you're investing in your health and well-being.

I only leak a bit and just when I'm running. Can I ignore this?

No, you can't ignore this. Well, you can, but our advice is that you shouldn't. Leaking is a sign that your body is not effectively managing what you're asking it to do. We can't replace our pelvic floor, so we need it to work for as long as possible, and the sooner you get on it the better – although, it's also never too late!

There is no way you'll master any of these exercises the first time you try them. It takes quite a bit of practice and coordination. Our top tip is to just stick with the process and don't worry too much if you're not getting it right at first. Like any skill that requires concentration and coordination, you'll improve with practice. Much as you do with all other aspects of your training, work on connecting, strengthening, coordinating and relaxing. This is just the beginning, but you'll be streets ahead of most if you can nail this and do it consistently, and your future self will thank you for making the effort.

We firmly believe that to maintain your long-term physical

health and well-being, you need to be doing a set of pelvic floor exercises every day. It's like doing basic drills and should be a part of your regular exercise programme. And the harder you train your body, the more you should be training your pelvic floor. Like every muscle in the body that needs to adapt, the pelvic floor needs to be stimulated and worked, mobilized and rested, and it needs to be coordinated. We look forward to the day that pelvic floor exercises are a feature of every training programme.

We know what the pelvic floor should do, we know that levels of knowledge around the pelvic floor are low,[6] and we know that a non-surgical approach to treatment involving doing pelvic floor exercises correctly and consistently, and/or being treated by a women's health physio works.[7] What we don't know is the impact this has on exercise performance – but we know enough to argue that we shouldn't be creating a culture where it's accepted that women are wetting themselves doing sport.

We think that every woman needs to have access to a specialized pelvic floor physiotherapist. We believe that women should have regular health checks to cover all aspects of their health, including a pelvic floor examination. In the UK, women's health physios are specifically trained to diagnose and treat pelvic floor symptoms. They are known by different terms around the world, and access to these specialists varies enormously depending on which country or region you live in. In the UK, you can see women's health physios on the NHS, but accessing them can be an issue as they are in high demand and tend to be available only to those with really extreme issues. France famously provides all post-natal women with *la rééducation périnéale*, in which all new mothers are given ten to twenty sessions of pelvic floor training. Many countries have private physios available and most health insurance companies will cover women's health physiotherapy, but, ironically, that's not always the case if the issues are birth-related.

If you have any of the issues listed above, or you're concerned about your pelvic floor in any way, then you must go and see your doctor. Even though they may not be able to offer you the detailed support you need, this is an important first step as they will be able to assess you, examine you and refer you to the necessary specialist. Our recommendation would be to also book in to see a women's health physio, who has the specific skills to treat the issues you're experiencing.

Pelvic floors are big business and we predict this is going to get bigger, with some exciting new technology and products coming on to the market. There are already some amazing products out there, but there are also some that at best do nothing and at worst can cause harm. There is no one treatment approach that suits all issues. There is no standard protocol or way of describing what to do or how to do it. Every woman is different, and if you have pelvic floor dysfunction, you need personalized care and not an off-the-shelf solution.

Pelvic floor golden rules:

- **Address the problem, don't hide it**
  Pads won't fix your pelvic floor, they mask the issue. They may keep you active which is great but do something about your symptoms, whether by seeing a professional or doing the exercises on pp. 102–4.

- **Work with an expert**
  Exercises work, spend your money on someone who can really support you and your issues.

- **Avoid gimmicks and gizmos**
  If you're experiencing pelvic floor issues that our basic and advanced exercises aren't fixing, your next step is to get a credible diagnosis. We don't recommend buying anything to put anywhere near your vagina unless a medical expert suggests it.

Toilet business

Problems with the pelvic floor can happen to any of us, but one of the reasons that pelvic floor dysfunction isn't talked about is because the common signs that it isn't working so well relate to wee and poo, which can be embarrassing topics, making it difficult for us to talk about this openly. We want to see that changed, so let's talk about what's normal for defecation and urination, because unless you know what's normal, you won't seek help when it isn't.

Bladders

Let's start with bladders. The bladder is a round sack that stores urine. As the urine drips into it, the bladder stretches and sends a signal to the brain to say you need to wee. This signal should be sent out when the bladder contains around 150ml of urine – but you don't need to go then; you can wait until you get a slightly stronger urge. You should be emptying your bladder five to seven times per day – every three hours or so – and it should take around eight to twelve seconds for you to produce 200–300ml of urine. This is news to most people; they can usually guess the number of loo visits but not the amount of urine produced.

It's perfectly possible to clock up twelve or more trips to the toilet a day. This is OK as a one-off, for example, on the day of a match or a race, nerves really do make you want to wee more often, and if you're also worried about leaking, you'll probably try and squeeze out every last drop before you begin your exercise.[8] But it's not OK to be going this often on a regular basis. If you're going this frequently, you may be hypersensitive to your bladder and your pelvic floor will not be getting 'trained' to hold a heavier bladder, which is important as we age. At night, you should be going to the toilet no more than once, so if you're going more frequently, this could be a sign of a weak pelvic floor or an over-enthusiastic hydration strategy (you're drinking too much!). The other extreme of little and often is never. Literally going at the start and the end of the day is not OK. Coaches, nurses, doctors and teachers often fall into this camp.

Baz recently worked with a retired physiotherapist who came to her because of a urinary-stress-incontinence issue. It wasn't until they had the 'how many times a day do you go to the loo' conversation that the woman had a light-bulb moment. She'd been proud of her 'iron bladder'; she'd never needed the loo, she told Baz. But after a discussion about how the bladder works, her issues started to make sense. Her whole life, her bladder was filling up so much that she had overstretched it. When she was younger it didn't matter, because the bladder bounced back, but as she aged and her connective tissue became less elastic, it stopped 'rebounding' and became floppy, which was what was causing her issues. She couldn't believe that what she thought of as a badge of honour – never needing a wee – was in fact causing her significant issues.

Here's a set of questions to ask yourself to recognize pelvic floor issues that may be impacting your bladder and health. Make sure you consult a healthcare professional if your answer is yes to any of the questions listed below.

- Do you limit fluid intake to try to prevent leaking?
- Do you wake up often when you're sleeping?
- Is there a conflict between hydration and sleep?
- How often do you think that you need a wee?
- Do certain foods irritate your bladder?
- Do you suffer from recurrent urinary tract infections?
- Do you go to the loo to empty your bladder, only to have to go again shortly after?
- Do you fully empty your bladder? If there's some retention, this can cause a small stagnant pool in your bladder, which can make you prone to infection.
- Do you have a small leak when you get up from the loo?

Bowels

Knowing what is normal, understanding our own bowel movements and taking action when things start to change is part of Dame Deborah James's legacy. She worked wonders in bringing bowels into the mainstream conversation in the UK with her mission to help people spot bowel cancer early.[9] The awareness she brought to the topic will not only save lives, it will also improve the health of many people as bowels can tell us so much about our bodies – including how our pelvic floor is doing. But given that we don't even want to talk about wetting ourselves, we certainly don't want to talk about being constipated or having such an overwhelming urge to poo that it's stopping us from doing what we love.

Let's start with some basics. Here's what's normal:

- emptying your bowels once or twice in twenty-four hours
- having a smooth, banana-shaped stool
- taking your time and not having to push – it should come out easily

Bowel issues can have many contributing factors, and the solution is often based on lifestyle. There will, of course, be times when medical support is necessary, but for most people the fix is pretty straightforward, even if it isn't easy.

Let's start with constipation. Firstly, no one should be constipated, and it is fixable. If you go fewer than three times a week, have hard stools or have to push to pass them, you're constipated. You may get really bad back pain as well, when stools build up over time. Being constipated isn't healthy, as it means you're not excreting toxins and your gut isn't balanced. It can also be a sign of a weak pelvic floor or of high levels of stress, anxiety or poor nutrition. Whatever the reason, the body is sending a pretty clear message that things are not OK and you need to pay attention. Your first port of call should be a doctor or alternative health specialist – someone who isn't just immediately going to prescribe a laxative – and who will sit with you for some time to try to work out what the triggers for your constipation could be. The solution may be really simple – drink more water and eat more vegetables – or it may be more complex, but there needs to be a holistic approach, and time should be taken to sort it out.

At the other end of the spectrum from constipation is having loose stools and, again, the causes of this can depend on a number of factors. You may even be experiencing both conditions – being constipated at some times and having loose stools at others. You may also have an underlying gut issue or medical concern. Again, we encourage you to talk to the right person – someone who can help you, and not just someone who can sympathize. Talk to a reputable health professional who has experience to support you with the changes you'll need to make.

Lastly, you may have bowel urges while out running, or just before your period or after having a coffee. Understanding more about why you're getting these urges, what your pattern is, the impact of certain foods or what happens at certain stages of your menstrual cycle, will help you piece together the right solution.

Bella

The first time I heard Baz speak about bowels was at an event in London, and I was blown away by all the information and tips that she gave. Believe it or not, many patients I see are preoccupied with their bowels and I think the older we get, the more obsessed with them we become. It is so important that we know our own normal bowel habits. Good bowel function is a sign of good health, and changes to our bowels can be a symptom of underlying disease. I had one patient who was really struggling with constipation and she often relied on laxatives to keep her bowels regular. I recommended she watch one of Baz's webinars, after which she made the simple but effective change of having a footstool to rest her feet on when opening her bowels. This was life-changing for her and she no longer relies on medication.

Here are some top tips for good bowel health.

1. Respond to your urge
   Once you feel the urge to poo, try to go within fifteen to twenty minutes, after which your body will stop sending cues to poo and you won't feel like going any more, even though the poo is still there. One problem is that we prefer to go at home, so if we get the urge when we're out, we tend to ignore it. But the poo needs to come out, and if we don't respond to our urges, the likelihood of becoming constipated is pretty high, which isn't a good thing at all when it comes to our pelvic floor.

2. Use a footstool
   Put your feet up on a toddler step to get your knees above your hips, lean forward, relax and let go – no pushing. This is the perfect pooing position! Leaning forwards is important for good propulsion: think of emptying your bowels back and down, not just down.

3. Don't strain
   It's very important not to strain as this can lead to other issues such as pelvic organ prolapse. If you're straining regularly, a women's health physio can improve your technique and teach you how to empty your bowels without straining, while supporting the pelvic floor.

4. Look at your poo

We're all used to looking at our urine to see if we're hydrated or not. Look at your poo as well, to see how it's formed, so you know what's normal for you.

The more information we have about how our bodies are functioning, the better. Having conversations about topics that have been shrouded in shame or secrecy for too long will destigmatize them, bring them out in the open and help everyone to learn more and check in with their habits. We understand that it may seem bizarre to be proposing that you talk more openly about your body – and especially your bladder and bowel habits – but be brave and give it a go. You'll be amazed at how much everyone will want to talk about theirs!

Baz

Many women come to me with constipation questions (I have a bit of a reputation for being the 'Poo Whisperer'!). One woman I worked with was a management consultant who told me that she only went for a poo once a week. I kid you not! She said she never had time to go and hated going anywhere other than at home, which was causing huge issues. I knew we had a lot of work to do, but the fix came quickly, and in fact I got a text from her one day, as she was travelling on the train into London with her husband, about how she'd got the urge (as usual) but instead of ignoring it (as usual), she went to the loo at the station. She was astounded to find everyone in there doing a poo. It was totally liberating for her and she felt so good about herself that she couldn't wait to tell me!

How to perfect your pelvic floor

If you do just one thing to improve your pelvic floor health, it should be to start doing pelvic floor exercises every day. If you're feeling more ambitious, here are a few other ideas.

- Don't let yourself get constipated – address this issue as and when it happens to avoid creating other health problems, including pelvic floor issues.
- Track your trips to the loo: understand your bladder and bowel habits and take action if you need to.
- Don't accept leaking as an 'oops' moment. Your pelvic floor should keep you dry. If it doesn't, it's not working properly, but you *can* do something about it. It's never too late.
- Have a low bar when asking for help. Let's change the seven-year statistic – the current amount of time it takes women to ask an expert for help with pelvic floor dysfunction.
- Think about your pelvic floor when you're on the gym floor – are you protecting or pulverizing your pelvic floor during your workouts? Can you fit your pelvic floor exercises into your gym routine?

Chapter 6

Supporting Your Breasts Well

We love rolling out a good statistic to get people interested in how important all areas of women's health are for sports performance. Whether we talk to world champions or weekend warriors, schoolgirls or veteran athletes, the one stat that people love, and continue to share, is that by wearing a well-fitting sports bra you may be able to achieve a 4% improvement in performance. To put this in context, if you wore an ill-fitting sports bra and raced a marathon against a clone of yourself who was wearing a well-fitting bra, the clone would finish a mile ahead of you.[1] A whole mile ahead, just because of a bra! And although this is a running example, no matter which sport or activity you do, if you are moving, your breasts are moving, and that has an influence on how your body performs.

Since 80% of women wear an ill-fitting bra,[2] that's a whole lot of women who could significantly improve their performance, comfort and enjoyment in sport for the cost of getting the right bra. Extraordinary. In this chapter we'll look at why the sports bra is one of your best wardrobe allies as an active woman, and just how you can ensure you've got the right bra with the best fit.

A bra is never a bad idea

Regardless of some of the myths that do the rounds on social media, or how good it feels to get your bra off at the end of the day, there is no evidence that wearing a bra is bad for any aspect of your health. Absolutely no research has shown that wearing a bra is bad for you. And getting yourself a great-fitting everyday bra, as well as a great-fitting sports bra, is a fantastic investment in your health and performance.

> ### Emma
>
> You know when Homer Simpson does something stupid and shouts 'Doh!' while slapping his forehead? Well, that was me when I realized that I had completely overlooked just how important sports bras and breast health were for active women, despite putting together what I had thought was a comprehensive campaign to support Olympic and Paralympic female athletes at the English Institute of Sport. I was at the University of Portsmouth delivering a presentation, when I mentioned that we had begun a strategic focus on the female athlete. At the end, Professor Joanna Wakefield-Scurr, who heads up a world-leading research group studying the biomechanics of the breast during sport, asked, 'I wonder whether our work in breast support would be of interest for your female athlete programme?' In that moment I realized I hadn't even considered breast support – we'd been focusing on the menstrual cycle, female-athlete injury, pelvic floor health . . . but not breasts and bras!
>
> That day at lunch, Jo and I decided we would get every Olympic and Paralympic female athlete into the best bra they'd ever had. We delivered educational workshops to

athletes, researched what they really wanted from a sports bra, and then worked with an amazing bra designer, Emily Roberts, to develop the ultimate sports bras, which were then professionally fitted on the athletes. I learned so much in that process, and just like all the areas we cover in this book, once you know the facts, you'll wonder why no one has ever told you this before. And if you're like me, every time you see an awesome woman pounding the pavements on her run, breasts bouncing rather than properly supported, you'll want to stop the car, run up to her and tell her too.

What's in a breast?

The female breast is a pretty unique structure because it has a relatively large mass with no muscle or bone to support it. If we look at our body, bones, muscles, ligaments and tendons all help keep our bits and bobs in place, but that's not true of the breast. It's a blob made up mostly of fatty tissue, with some connective tissue that provides a small amount of structural support from inside the breast mass. This connective tissue is called Cooper's ligaments, although ligaments is a very misleading label because elsewhere in the body ligaments attach from bone to bone, as in the knee's anterior cruciate ligament. The third component of the breast is glandular tissue – the functional bit, made up of the milk glands and ducts, which are used for breastfeeding.

We have muscle and bone in the vicinity of the breast – our ribs sit behind the breast tissue, providing a foundation on which they rest, and our pectoral muscles sit on top of the ribs – but neither actually holds the breast securely in place. Inside the breast are thin bands of connective tissue – Cooper's ligaments – which play a role in supporting the shape of the breast. But this connective tissue isn't very strong and that leaves the skin as the breast tissue's main supporting structure. Our skin reaches its most healthy and elastic state during our mid-twenties, and from then on it's quite literally downhill, as the skin loses its natural elasticity. This is what causes breasts to sag over time, as the skin holding the breast in place is stretched.[3]

But researchers in breast health also suggest that a repeated bouncing motion of the breast can lead to irreparable damage to the skin. When we move – whether it's walking, running, cycling or dancing – our breasts move (and bigger breasts move more), particularly if they are poorly supported by an ill-fitting bra. They can move in all directions, and they move most when the activity is high-impact, such as running and jumping. Research conducted on women running bare-breasted on a treadmill (ouch!) in a lab proved that each breast can move up to 20cm, and moves about 15cm for the average-breast-size woman doing jogging or an aerobics-type activity. Given that each breast typically weighs about half a kilogram it's perhaps not surprising that movement of that magnitude can cause the skin to stretch beyond its natural elastic range, from which it cannot bounce back.

Baz

A mum friend told me her daughter had stopped going to swim club before school because the other girls were teasing her about her breasts being different sizes. This breaks my heart, not just because it's girls being mean to each other instead of supporting each other, but because the lack of education about what's normal and what's not would have been really helpful here. Knowing that most women have uneven-size breasts, and that the size difference can appear most dramatically during puberty and tends to become imperceivable over time, might have been enough to make that swimmer less amusing to her peers, or more confident that her breast development was normal.

A pain in the breast

One of the most common problems the breast poses for active women – and we are talking about healthy breasts here – is breast pain. Researchers have found that breast pain is experienced by over 50% of women.[4] Most commonly the pain is experienced cyclically, as a menstrual cycle symptom, where breasts are sore at certain times of the month. Other breast pain can be non-cyclical, so not related to your menstrual cycle, but presenting as intermittent or permanent breast pain (if this applies to you, please see your doctor; it's likely benign but needs checking). The third type of breast pain, and the most newly acknowledged, is exercise-induced breast pain, where the movement of the breast caused by exercise is painful. Exactly why our breasts hurt during exercise is not yet known. Researchers are unsure whether it's the amount of movement, or its frequency or speed. Regardless of its cause, breast pain during exercise is common among active women and was reported by 63% of athletes in an Australian study, with 44% saying that the breast pain interfered with their performance.[5] Another study, undertaken at the 2012 London Marathon, found that 32% of the participants had experienced breast pain, and 17% said it had impacted how much they could train for the event.[6]

Breast enlargement and breast pain is also a very common symptom in the premenstrual phase (experienced by about 50% of women), and you may need a more supportive bra at this time of your cycle, or you might try to find a sports bra with good adjustability so that it can accommodate changing breast size and still give the best support. Breast pain shouldn't be a barrier to exercise or impact the quality of your training, because in most cases there is a simple solution: getting the right style and fit of sports bra.

Now, when we say a simple solution, that's assuming you actually know what type of sports bra you need and that you know how to ensure it fits really well. Yet these are things we're not taught, which moves this simple solution into the realm of unknown possibility. To set that straight, we'll cover how to find the right style and fit of sports bra later in this chapter.

When your D-cup overfloweth

If movement of the breast during exercise causes problems, then bigger breasts are a bigger problem, because large breasts move the most during exercise. Large breasts are defined as D-cup and above, and it's from this size onwards that sports bra design often changes to support larger, heavier breasts during exercise. University of Wollongong researchers found that larger-breasted women often didn't know how to find the right bra, so they ended up in an ill-fitting or wrong style of sports bra, which meant that during exercise their breasts moved a lot more, which increased their discomfort, which in turn led them to do less physical activity.[7] This lack of exercise often meant these women put on weight, which increased their breast mass further, meaning their bra was even less suited to the job. They were stuck in a perpetual big-breast, bad-bra situation.

There's also evidence that breast pain occurs more frequently in women who have larger breasts; movement and pain have been identified as the two main reasons that larger-breasted women do less physical activity. A 2018 study found that women with large breasts spent 37% less time participating in physical activity than women with small breasts, particularly doing less vigorous-intensity physical activity.[8] A high percentage of these women directly attributed the intensity of the physical activity they performed to their breast size – poor breast support is actually stopping some of us from being active. The authors of the research concluded their paper with some advice that 'women with larger breasts should select activities that are more appropriate for women with large breasts, such as water-based activities'. While that's well-intentioned advice, it goes against our core values at The Well HQ. A lack of information about how best to support their breasts shouldn't be the reason women stop doing exercise or activities they love. There is information available that means your breast size doesn't have to dictate whether you can or can't be active and you mustn't feel that your body is holding you back from doing what you love.

The notion that big-breasted women can't be sporty is perpetuated by the myth that all elite athletes are flat-chested. It's true, some elite athletes have small breasts. And some don't – it's as simple as that. Breast size is not a defining feature of successful athletes. We've worked with elite athletes who have breast sizes varying from 32–44 inches and cup sizes AA–J.

However, larger-breasted athletes often have to work harder to find the right bra. Serena Williams, the awesome tennis legend, has openly shared her underwhelming experiences of sports bras as a larger-breasted athlete, saying that she couldn't find a bra for her size that also had the support she needed for doing such high-impact activities. When she did come across a brand and style that she loved, she stuck with it, despite the brand only being available in Australia for the first fifteen years after she discovered it. She'd buy fifty bras each year she went to the Australian Open, ensuring she never had to be without one, wearing the same model of bra for every match for two decades. There is no one-size-fits-all bra solution for every active woman, so what works for Serena might not work for you, but it's always useful to have recommendations from people who have really put their kit to the test, so ask those in your circle who regularly exercise for their top tips and when you find your perfect bra, spread the word.

When your D-cup is half empty

We want to emphasize the need for good breast support during sport for smaller-breasted women and adolescents too – the mechanics of your body can be constantly changing due to breast movement, no matter how small the mass of your breast. A sports bra is an essential bit of kit for when girls and women are moving their bodies. It should be a required item on PE and kit lists for schools. All the performance impacts of wearing ill-fitting bras that we'll talk about in the next sections – such as shortened stride-length, impaired breathing or greater energy requirements – apply to all breast sizes, including women with smaller breasts. And movement during sport and activity can still cause damaging skin strains in women with A- and B-cup sizes, eventually leading to breast sag and/or stretch marks.[9]

Not all breasts were created equal

Did you know that 94% of women have breast asymmetry – where one breast is larger or a different shape than the other? (It's more common for the left breast to be larger, in case you were wondering.[10]) There's a scientific reason why that's important to know. Breast asymmetry leads to asymmetrical movement of breasts during exercise, and when a woman's bra doesn't fit both of her breasts well, it can lead to more movement in one breast, which can lead to pain and discomfort. For women with breast asymmetry, it's important to select encapsulation sports bras, where both the shoulder straps and underband are adjustable, as they can be altered to support each breast effectively.

A bra for everyone

Depending on your breast size, your body shape and what type of exercise you do, there will be a best bra style for you. Your priority when looking for a sports bra should be decreasing breast motion and increasing comfort (the pretty colour or bad-ass strap design come bottom of the list – sorry).

Sports bras come in three styles:

Encapsulation

This type of sports bra is made of sturdy, supportive fabric, designed so that each breast is supported separately. There is usually a back fastening on the underband, and you can adjust both the shoulder straps and the underband. Sometimes encapsulation sports bras are underwired. Research has shown this type of sports bra is the best for reducing breast movement in large-breasted women (a D-cup and above).

Compression (aka crop tops)

This type of bra compresses, or squashes, the breast tissue against your chest, making both breasts form a single unit. By doing this, the bra actually now has to cope with double the breast mass, compared with a bra that supports each breast separately. This is one of the reasons crop tops are not recommended for bigger breasts (larger than a D-cup) – there's just too much breast tissue to deal with once it's all squashed together in one lump![11] However, squashing the breast tissue closer to your torso re-positions the centre of mass of the breast closer to your body, which reduces the forces acting through the breast, which in turn reduces movement of the breast. That said, the crop-top bra is usually made from one piece of stretchy material, and since it has no fastenings it must be put on over the head. Because of this, the lifespan of crop tops is not as long as other types of bra, as all this stretching to get it on and off over time loosens the underband and therefore impacts the supportiveness of the bra.

Combination

As the name suggests, this bra design is a combination of both of the above sports bra types, usually comprising two separate cups to encapsulate each breast, covered with an external layer to compress the breast tissue – a double whammy. These types of bras are good for supporting large-breasted women, reducing breast movement and alleviating breast pain more effectively than the other styles individually.

Different styles of sports bra provide different levels of support

When Emma worked on the sports bra project for elite athletes, the athletes were asked in advance what style of bra they would prefer. Interestingly, prior to the fitting, the majority of athletes opted for a compression-style bra over encapsulation. Following the fittings in both bras, and advice from the expert bra fitter, 30% of the athletes opted to change to an encapsulation bra. These were athletes who lived every day in a sports bra and thought they had found the best type of bra for them and their sport – yet so many of them found that there was a more optimal bra fit and style out there for them.

As well as different designs of bra, you can use the features of the sports bra itself to ensure that you are really getting the best support from it. When looking at a prospective bra, bear in mind the following:

- **Shoulder straps** that are wide, padded and adjustable will help you to get a great fit. A racer-back or shoulder-strap design doesn't make a difference to support levels but can be a personal preference.
- **A higher neckline** will improve the bounce-reduction qualities of the bra.
- **An adjustable underband** will ensure the best fit.
- **Some padding** will help reduce breast bounce.
- **Underwire** can improve the supportiveness of the bra.

Getting the best fit

Most women will be familiar with a bra fitting that happens in the changing room of a department store or lingerie shop, which involves a lovely shop assistant and a tape measure. The trouble with the tape-measure approach is that it originated before bras were made out of stretchy or adjustable material, and in some places bra fitters still compensate for the historically rigid fabric by adding on inches to the exact measurement to allow for room to breathe. However, modern bra fabric and design is completely different now from when they were first introduced, in the 1850s when they were made of wood and whalebone sewn into material. Plus, having someone measure your size is one thing, but it leaves many women assuming that all bras in this size will be the perfect fit, which simply isn't the case.

A tape measure is still a good place to start, as you'll see from our measuring guide – it gives you an idea of your underband and cup size, but then it's important to use the five-step fit criteria to check whether your bra fits you really well.

Measuring your size

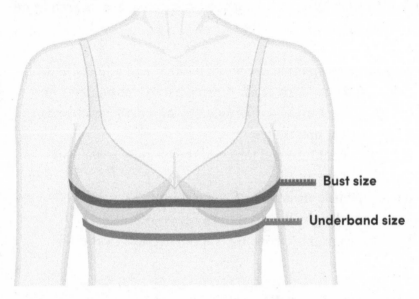

Bust size

Underband size

Where to measure your bust and underband size

1. First measure under your breasts, around your rib cage, to get your underband measurement, in inches.
2. Then measure around the fullest part of your bust, usually across the nipple line, again in inches.
3. Subtract your underband measurement from your bust measurement, then use the table below to convert that difference, in inches, into your cup size.

Difference between underband and cup measurements (inches)	+1	+2	+3	+4	+5	+6	+7	+8	+9
Cup size	A	B	C	D	DD	E	F	FF	G

For example, if your underband measured 32in and round your bust measured 36in, there is a difference of 4in between underband and bust. The table shows that +4 is a D cup. Your bra size is 32 D.

Sizes may vary

We all know what it's like: thinking you know what size you are, buying a size 14 top from a particular shop and being delighted with the fit, then the same day trying on a size 14 top from a different shop and finding it's too small – go figure. Different shops, different brands, different designs of clothes can be different sizes, despite having the same number on the label. The same is true for bras, so even when you think you know your bra size, it's possible that in different bra brands, or even in sports bras vs your everyday bras, you won't be the same size. So, instead of focusing on the size or the brand, focus more on the fit. Fit is the foundation of breast support. Consider how much time some of us spend on choosing the right trainers; some might even use the special treadmills in running shops to measure our foot-strike, to see what type of support our foot needs. Imagine if we spent as much time and did our due diligence on getting the right fit and type of bra.

The best way to check that you're in the right size of sports bra is by working through this five-point fitting guide.

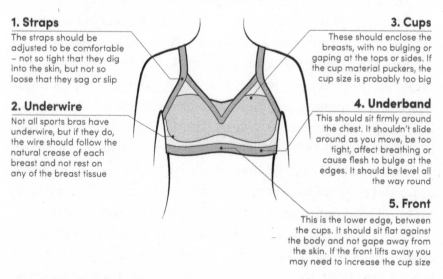

1. Straps
The straps should be adjusted to be comfortable – not so tight that they dig into the skin, but not so loose that they sag or slip

2. Underwire
Not all sports bras have underwire, but if they do, the wire should follow the natural crease of each breast and not rest on any of the breast tissue

3. Cups
These should enclose the breasts, with no bulging or gaping at the tops or sides. If the cup material puckers, the cup size is probably too big

4. Underband
This should sit firmly around the chest. It shouldn't slide around as you move, be too tight, affect breathing or cause flesh to bulge at the edges. It should be level all the way round

5. Front
This is the lower edge, between the cups. It should sit flat against the body and not gape away from the skin. If the front lifts away you may need to increase the cup size

Five-point fitting guide

The perfect match

Many of us don't do the same type of activity every time we work out, and that means our breasts might need a different type of support from one day to the next. If your training ranges from yoga to Zumba, you might want different types of breast support for these activities – perhaps a highly supportive, structured encapsulation bra for your exercise to fast music, but a softer, less supportive bra for mat work. If you only have one sports bra, make sure it supports the highest-impact activity that you do.

Doubling up

We've all done it or know someone who has: wearing two bras to exercise. Women do this for many reasons: because they are wearing the wrong style of bra, usually a compression bra that doesn't provide adequate support on its own; or they don't want to buy an expensive new bra when surely wearing the two old ones they do have can give enough support. We say no. Two old bras won't do the job. Furthermore, it actually increases the chance of chafing or pain from a poor fit, twice over. There is an amazing bra out there for you and it comes in a one-pack. Do your research, look at whether the brand has been tested for its effectiveness in reducing breast motion, use our fitting and style guides to find the right type and size for you, and don't stop until you get what you need. It's not an indulgence for you to spend money on a well-fitting bra; it's in your best interests, and in the long-term best interests of your breasts. Think of how much we spend on our running shoes and leggings then think of your sports bra as another essential bit of workout gear, not just a nice-to-have. Sports bra brands now offer excellent help on their websites to guide you to the design that will work best for you, and some even have live chat functions to help you choose. Some women say they won't know that a bra doesn't fit well until they've been for a run in it. This is usually because they haven't assessed the fit properly when they tried it on, checking all of the five points. Doing some star jumps in a changing room is a good way to test motion control – they're one of the exercises that causes the most breast movement.

Bad bras, bad bras, whatcha gonna do?

We've established that poorly supported breasts move and that movement can cause pain and discomfort that can impact how well you can train, or whether you train at all. But if your breasts aren't bothering you, is there any reason to pay attention to all this talk of getting better breast support? Yes – because as you now know, if you're not in a well-fitted sports bra that's designed for the type of activity you're doing, then your breasts are literally slowing you down. It doesn't even matter what type of exercise you do – whether you run, row, kayak, play tennis or golf, go to the gym, hike mountains or chase after kids. If you're moving, your breasts are moving. And unless you have them in a well-fitted sports bra, that breast movement will hamper your performance.

Friends of ours at the University of Portsmouth have done a series of studies looking at how sporting performance is impacted by poor breast support. In their research they compared women exercising in an everyday bra versus a well-fitted sports bra. Here's what they found.

- **Exercise is easier in a good bra**
  When asked to rate their effort during the same exercise, women reported that it was easier when wearing a well-fitted sports bra than when wearing an unsupportive bra.[12] Let's just repeat that: a good bra makes exercise easier. Who doesn't want that?

- **Exercise in an ill-fitting bra might increase your risk of injury**
  When breasts move during exercise, they don't just bounce up and down (which accounts for 50% of their movement during running), they also move side to side (25% of the movement) and forward and back (the other 25%). The forces caused by these movements are transferred right through our body to the ground during running and could become a risk-factor for injury.[13]

- **Ill-fitting bras make you more tired during training**
  When running with poor breast support, your upper-body muscles are more activated.[14] It's thought this is to try to counteract the effect the breast movement is having on your body. Activating more muscles uses more energy, so the cost of breast movement might be that you get tired quicker than if you were wearing a well-fitted bra.

- **Breast movement during exercise can interfere with how we breathe**
  Research shows that breathing frequency – our breaths per minute – is decreased when breast support is poor, and that women hold their breath for longer as if to brace themselves against the movements of their breasts.[15] We know that breathing is strongly linked to the pace of exercise: how hard we breathe is one of the signals to the brain of how hard we're working. Altering breathing frequency can make exercise feel harder, and mucking up our natural breathing patterns by having an unsupportive bra also means that we might not be getting as much air, including precious oxygen, throughout our exercise, which can make us get tired quicker.

- **You cover less ground with each stride in a bad bra**
  The statistic mentioned earlier – that we lose the equivalent

of a mile over a marathon in an ill-fitting bra – is influenced by the fact that stride-length decreases when our breasts aren't fully supported during running.[16] Even a small shortening of stride-length can, over the course of 5km, 10km or a marathon, add up to quite a significant amount of lost ground, not because you aren't fit enough, but because your body is trying to adapt to the movement of your poorly supported breasts by shortening your stride.

A blow to the breast

Something we don't talk about much is breast injuries. These might be contact breast injuries that sports players get during a game of rugby or basketball or during combat sports. Breast injury is more common than previously realized: in a study of 500 elite female athletes from forty-six different sports, 36% reported experiencing breast injuries and 21% thought that their breast injury negatively affected their performance.[17] Pain associated with breast injury is one thing, but injury to the breast tissue can also cause 'dead fat necrosis' (damaged or dead breast tissue) which can lead to lumps in the breast. These lumps can be mistaken for breast cancer and might therefore require a biopsy to exclude cancer. Injury to the breast does not increase a woman's risk of breast cancer, but because of the lumps that it can leave behind, it can cause unnecessary worry and invasive procedures.[18] Frustratingly, body armour in sport is usually designed for men and is not styled to accommodate and protect breasts at all.[19] However, some solutions have been developed for women in recent years, designed to protect breast tissue and prevent breast injury, including inserts for sports bras and female-fit padded vests.[20]

Women might also experience breast injury in the form of rubbing and chafing. Poor bra fit is usually to blame, so just as we wouldn't accept our trainers continuously giving us blisters, we shouldn't accept breast injury being a normal part of exercising, and should search for a better fit to stop the rub.

Emma

It was fortunate that my husband was part of my support crew for an ultra-distance race I did with two male colleagues. We were running 100km along the South Downs Way, a beautiful countryside trail in Sussex. Every 10km there was a chance to meet your support crew, top up water bottles, grab some food and pop on a dry t-shirt. The only thing that was different about my pit-stop routine versus the guys' was that mine also involved my husband scooping enormous quantities of Vaseline into his hands and spreading the stuff under my bra. I was suffering very badly from chafing around the underband and under my arms, so much so that sometimes it stopped me training, and I wore blister plasters on hotspots every time I ran. I wasn't as well educated in the world of breast support in those days, and I wore two bras, neither of which, in retrospect, fitted that well. The result was friction and skin injuries that were best helped by ensuring I had lubricant between the bra and my skin. It worked OK for the 100km race, but having my own personal lubricant applicator running around after me wasn't really a long-term option. Eventually, however, just like Serena Williams, I found my bra-for-life.

It's not just blows to the breasts or chafing that can cause damage for active women. The effect of a poorly fitting bra can also cause musculoskeletal problems in the back, shoulder and neck, which manifest as tension, tightness and pain. Physiotherapists even use bras as a way to treat postural problems to relieve neck and back pain, and to improve posture. Shoulder straps that are too tight can also dig into the skin, leaving permanent furrows, and compression of nerves, which can lead to tingling or numbness in the arm and hand. This is often a problem experienced by women with larger breasts, who try and prevent breast movement by tightening the straps of their bra and end up supporting most of the weight of their breast tissue through the straps, with not enough support provided by a well-fitting underband (which is where the majority of support for your breasts should come from).

Points to remember for the best breast support

- Find the right type of sports bra for supporting your breast size in the activities you like to do. Then make sure it fits you properly.
- You don't have to spend a fortune on a sports bra. Proper support and a good fit are more important than the name on the label.
- Don't let breast-related pain hold you back. Find a bra that supports your breasts well enough so that it minimizes breast, back and shoulder pain.

Chapter 7

Bodies that Move Well

In March 2020, the UK government ordered all gyms and sports clubs to close, as the country went into its first Covid-19 lockdown. Despite exercise being one of the only permitted reasons to leave your home, physical activity levels decreased during the lockdowns of 2020 and 2021, and sedentary behaviour increased.[1] In women, this situation was compounded by childcare, homeschooling and housework duties, which are usually three times greater for women than men but during the Covid lockdowns increased further, so that women were spending over thirty hours per week on childcare alone.[2] No wonder they didn't have time to pull on the Lycra and expend some energy; women were, quite literally, exhausted by the burden of care they took on during the pandemic.

The consequence of this lockdown hiatus in exercising was an exponential increase in injuries as people returned to their preferred method of being active – whether it was finding time for a run once the kids were finally back in school or returning to the netball court or gym as leisure centres opened up again. In elite sport, where injury is well documented, injury rates increased threefold before athletes even played their first match.[3] It wasn't just elite athletes who fell foul of returning to play a little too eagerly. At that time, the three of us were supporting England Netball with its 'Back to Netball' campaign, and we were hearing similar stories from girls and women across the country whose new season ended before it really began, after they picked up injuries in the first few sessions back on court.

Zero to hero, and back again

As women, we often expose ourselves to this type of zero-to-hero scenario, but not usually with a pandemic lockdown involved. We have a notorious all-or-nothing approach to healthy habits like diet and exercise. Yet this type of yo-yo-ing, particularly when it comes to exercise, is a recipe for sustaining an injury.

As simple as it sounds, some of the best progress can be made in health and fitness by consistently doing some exercise at your current fitness level, and then gradually and safely raising the bar. Showing up and moving consistently is a far more sustainable approach than spending chunks of time not doing any physical activity and then deciding to embark upon a new five-day-a-week HIIT regime. In fact, research suggests that the likelihood of you reaching your goal (whether that's a parkrun or a podium finish) is increased seven times if you train regularly and consistently, rather than spending time ill, injured or not motivated to exercise.[4] Staying in one piece, not missing workouts, and taking your opportunities to move, are the secret sauce for getting healthier and fitter.

Women seem to have the odds stacked against them when it comes to building up consistency in their training or exercise regime.

Reasons

1. For many women, menstrual cycle symptoms can affect their motivation to move, or the quality of our workout, for many days each month. If you are losing three to five

days per month of training because of symptoms, that's sixty days per year!

2. Women often have more competing demands on their time. It's hard to fit in that early-morning run if you have children and you have to get them out of the door for school; or you may forgo your basketball practice to take them to theirs; or you have to add the cost of childcare to the cost of your class and it just becomes prohibitively expensive.

3. Women are up to six times more likely to suffer a joint injury than men, which means time out of the movement and exercise you enjoy, so you can recover.[5]

Solutions

1. Now that you have the strategies to deal with menstrual cycle symptoms, implement them to regain those lost days of exercise.

2. We totally get it; as three working mums, we, too, navigate this struggle daily. But we can't emphasize enough the need to prioritize time for your body and your mind.

3. Warm up before and cool down after exercise and be mindful of your technique to ensure you don't put undue stress on your joints that can lead to injury.

We know it's not easy. It took Emma about eight years to reset her relationship with exercise after having her first child. After pursuing audacious goals for marathons and ultra-endurance events throughout her twenties and early thirties, once her children arrived it took many years of trying different approaches to working out and moving to find activities that were both satisfying and sustainable.

It's such an individual challenge. For some, it's about finding a free online workout that you enjoy, that you might be able to do when your kids sleep, or which they can join in with. For others, home workouts just don't hit the spot, but popping the baby in the buggy or putting the kids on the scooter, then power-walking or jogging around the park, feels a great way to move. But for many women, it's about giving yourself permission to prioritize your body, your mental and physical health, and to feel OK about taking thirty minutes out of your working day to work out, on your own, child-free if you're a mum. Because many of us, particularly mothers, feel guilty about using our spare time – such as when the children are at school, childcare or a playdate – for ourselves. We cram that time with extra work, household chores or other responsibilities and we don't realize that one of the most productive, beneficial things we can do for our long-term health and well-being is to move in a way that we truly enjoy. And don't underestimate how impactful your children seeing you exercising will be on their future behaviour. They will see taking time to exercise as a normal, import-ant part of life. That's an amazing gift to give them!

This is a public service announcement

We'd like to delve into women's injuries in a bit more depth because there's simply not enough priority given to informing women about their injury risk and what to do about it, yet every day we meet women who aren't doing the sport or activity they love because they suffered an injury that now prevents them from taking part.

How many of you have been in a fitness class, or a group warm-up, and heard the generic warning chanted by trainers, coaches and fitness instructors not to let our knees go over our toes when doing exercises like lunges? This rule of thumb is intended to establish good technique and prevent injury. But there should be a second part to that public service announcement that we never hear, and which should go something like this:

'For women in the group, pay special attention to your technique: don't let your knees cave in; engage your hamstrings, glutes and core rather than just relying on your quads – because you're much more likely to suffer a knee injury than men, and these are the things you can do to stop that happening.'

While this may dampen the atmosphere of the BodyPump class or CrossFit warm-up, it's a very important message. Anterior cruciate ligament (ACL) injury has been referred to as an epidemic in women's sport.[6] The ACL is the ligament that connects your thigh bone to your shin bone. This tough, elastic band of tissue runs diagonally through the inside of the knee and stabilizes the joint. An ACL injury happens when the way your leg moves stretches the ligament too much, and it tears or completely ruptures. This can happen when you make a rapid change of direction or the knee gets twisted while running, turning, jumping or landing. And figures show that women are up to six times more likely to suffer a non-contact ACL injury than men.[7] The 'non-contact' bit means that it's not caused by colliding with others or tripping over someone else's hockey stick; it happens with no contact at all, just from the forces of the movement of your body. The bad news is that of those who do suffer an ACL injury, 45% never compete again and 35% do not meet their previous level of athleticism. Up to half of 15–30-year-olds show signs of osteoarthritis just a decade after having an ACL injury,[8] which is much higher than the average prevalence of 7% in 18–44-year-olds.[9]

It's not just ACL injuries that are more common in women. Across the body, women are more at risk of joint injury than men.[10] The ankle is another joint where injuries frequently occur – about two times more often in women – and the shoulder, too, is more commonly injured in women than in men.[11]

Due to the clearly devastating impact of joint injury on women's short-term participation in sport and exercise, and on their lifelong relationship with the activities they love, we really believe that awareness of, and protection against, this injury risk should be instilled in active women from a young age, and that it becomes an important consideration in coaching and training women across their lifespan. If girls and young women were taught PE and coached in ways that targeted and mitigated this risk, it's possible we could prevent many injuries in women doing sport. The increased risk in females is thought only to occur after puberty, since equal numbers of ligament sprains occur in girls and boys before adolescence but girls have higher rates immediately after their growth spurt and into maturity.[12] We still don't fully understand why women are at such an increased risk of joint injury, particularly at the knee (that's the gender data gap), but, having said that, in the last decade there has been important progress made in what we understand about potential risk factors and what we can do about them.

The thigh bone's connected to the hip bone . . . Now shake dem skeleton bones!

One risk factor for ACL injury relates to the anatomical differences between men and women. Women generally develop wider hips than males (because of our amazing childbearing capabilities), and this leads to a greater 'Q angle' – or quadriceps angle, which is the angle formed between the quadriceps muscles of the thigh and the patellar tendon of the knee – which is up to five degrees greater in women.

This wider angle has been linked to increased knee pain in women and to women's greater risk of ACL injury because it affects how females land from jumping movements or how they change in direction while running.[13] When we land or push off, the knee tends to cave in to what we call a valgus position, and

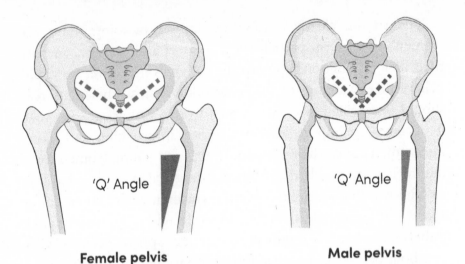

Female pelvis   **Male pelvis**

Q angle showing the 5-degree variation between women and men

this puts a lot of angular stress on the knee joint, which at best causes pain, and at worst is a contributing factor to injury at the knee joint.[14] Research has also shown that women's knees tend to cave inwards and that women tend to land jumps on their whole foot with a straighter knee, which means they have to absorb greater force than men, who land on their toes and then bend their knees to cushion the landing. Combine that greater force going through the knee joint with poor technique, causing that force to impact the joint at the wrong angle, and you start to see why the knee joint in women is so susceptible to injury. While we can't do anything about our skeleton, we can do something about the way we move, by training our jump-landing, balance, running and changing-direction techniques.

When you land from jumps, or you squat or lunge, make sure your knees don't cave inwards, that your knee doesn't pass too far over the toe, you bend your knees at impact to land softly and your knees and feet point in the same direction,[15] as shown in the following diagram.

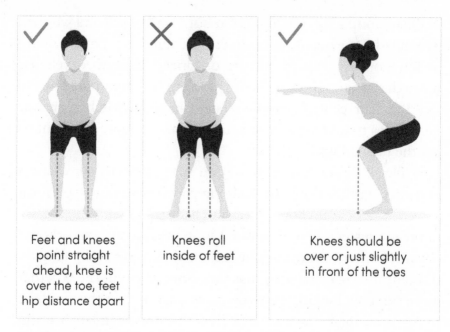

| Feet and knees point straight ahead, knee is over the toe, feet hip distance apart | Knees roll inside of feet | Knees should be over or just slightly in front of the toes |

Good technique when landing can help reduce injury risk

No one likes an over-active quad

Muscle strength and muscle imbalance are further risk factors in women when it comes to knee-joint injury. Women tend to be stronger in their quadriceps (the big muscle at the front of your leg) than in their glutes (the powerful muscles in your bottom) and hamstrings (the muscles at the back of your thigh), so the quads tend to take over what these other muscles should be doing during exercise.[16] This is known as 'quad dominance' and it's bad news for the knee joint because, during exercise like running, we need strong quads to straighten the knee and help to flex the foot forward, and then strong hamstrings and glutes to bend the knee and help to pull the leg backward, all while keeping our knee stable. The muscle groups should work together, switching on and off as we move through our stride. When they don't, usually because one is strong and the other is weak, the knee joint is at greater risk of injury.

Quad dominance is common in both active men and women, particularly in runners, who don't do enough strength training or hill work to balance out the quadricep strength developed through running. In women, the problem is compounded by the fact that our central nervous system happily switches on our quadriceps to deal with most situations and is more reluctant to get the hamstrings involved.[17]

While all this quadricep activation contributes to our chances of damaging the knee joint, it also impacts our ability to perform as well. By not letting our glutes and hamstrings get a look in, we miss out on some serious power. Our glutes are our powerhouse when it comes to moving our legs, and they are really fatigue-resistant too, which means that they don't tire quickly. Whether we're running, lunging or jumping, we may not get the most out of our movements unless we address this muscle imbalance and learn to switch on the right muscles at the right time with good technique and, at first, lots of concentration. This takes practice and can be done with conditioning exercises like squats, clams and glute bridges, which are well worth building into your regular training regime.

Resilient to the core

A common scenario is to take up an activity such as walking, running, cycling or netball and to spend all your workout time doing that particular activity or sport. In fact, this approach is really counterproductive when it comes to building injury resilience. It's called 'specificity' – when all your training is designed around one specific movement, game or sport. This approach to training makes our body very good at moving in these set ways, but doesn't build overall strength, mobility and stability. A whole-body conditioning approach gives us the stability to move with good technique, the strength to hold form when we are getting tired, and the mobility to cope with uneven terrain on a hike, or a sudden change of direction on the pitch. All of these things have the potential to cause injury if our whole body isn't conditioned to help out when it's needed during movement. This is why we see rowers rock climbing, rugby players learning to dance and netballers doing Pilates: it's a whole-body approach to building strong, resilient women. This means that even as a runner or a cyclist, upper-body and core work are an important part of your conditioning, as well as training all-important leg muscles. Research shows that having strength, flexibility and stability through your trunk and core will reduce injury even in your knees and ankles.[18]

Myth-buster: 'My menstrual cycle injured me!'

There have been a growing number of articles in newspapers about the link between the menstrual cycle and injury – so much so that, sometimes, when we talk to sportswomen, they tell us they're nervous about doing certain training sessions or playing matches at certain times of their cycle. We've even had physios and coaches asking whether they should not select players because of where they will be in their cycle at the time of their match. Let's get one thing straight: there's no future world we would design that means that on some days of the month we're wrapping women up in cotton wool and telling them not to move! The goal should be to understand what's happening in a woman's body and then to understand what it takes to make sure that thing doesn't cause her any problems.

As previously mentioned, there is a known link between oestrogen and joint stability. High oestrogen levels can loosen our joints,[19] which theoretically might make us more prone to injury at times in the cycle when oestrogen is high.[20] Some research has found that knee laxity can be greater just before ovulation, when oestrogen peaks.[21] However, we don't have enough reliable research on injury – as opposed to joint laxity – within particular times of the cycle to be sure if this theory actually plays out for active women. More research is needed to show whether there are other points in the cycle that are hotspots for injury: is it just when oestrogen is high prior to ovulation, or also when oestrogen rises again in the second half of the cycle?

It's certainly never going to be as simple as saying that all women are more likely to be injured at a certain time of the cycle. There are so many factors that can contribute to injury, and no one thing in isolation will be the cause of an injury. These factors may be physical, psychological, emotional or social, and they can all layer on top of each other to lead to an injury.[22] Take the woman who was up all night with a sick child turning up to hockey practice the following evening after a long day's work, tired, still worried about her child, playing on a second-rate surface because the men's first team got the nice pitch, not having eaten anything since lunch: the training session turns out to be a tough one, making her even more tired and leading her to lose some form in her running technique, and as she changes direction quickly to intercept the ball, her knee 'pops' – and she's torn her ACL. Women aren't buckling at the knees because their oestrogen is high. It may be possible that our hormones are another factor we can add to this list of things that create a perfect storm for injury, but we simply don't know for sure yet whether cycle hormones make that list.

When Emma worked with some of the world's best physios for Olympic and Paralympic athletes and posed the question of whether we should be worried about menstrual cycle hormones causing injury, their response was unanimous: rather than waiting to find out whether your oestrogen peak is the reason for your downfall, the best approach is always a proactive one. If you can make yourself more resilient, then your body will be able to withstand the stresses and strains of any activities you do because it has strength, agility, coordination and muscle balance that outweigh the effect of high oestrogen. All of these things are within your control, and you can start work on them now to protect yourself against injury.

Before we dispel the myth of the menstrual cycle and injury completely, it's worth adding that although the research doesn't show a solid link between the menstrual cycle and injury, we've seen athletes who are on the physio or massage table more at certain times of their cycle too often for it to be a mere coincidence. In these women, cycle hormones might have – as the science suggests – affected the laxity of their joints. Slightly less stable joints in the hip or the knee might also have a knock-on effect and cause a niggle in the back or a tight hamstring.

As for these athletes, knowing where you're at in your cycle can help you work out whether niggles or pain are related to your cycle. You can share this information with your physio or healthcare practitioner to help them identify possible causes. Depending on the day you're at in your cycle, you can develop an approach that takes this into consideration, like a particular taping or massage technique, or incorporate things into your warm-up, such as skill- and agility-work, to really switch on your neuromuscular system, or simply be extra vigilant about your technique at this time. As with all approaches to exercise, a consistent, long-term approach that addresses the range of risk factors that women are particularly prone to will give you a more injury-resilient body. It's not a quick fix, but it will pay dividends.

Reducing your injury risk

The best thing about knowledge is that it gives you power. You're not at the mercy of your biological sex, and that's never truer than when it comes to stamping out your increased risk of injury as a woman. Though we can't change the anatomy of our skeleton, we can change most of the other things that might put us at risk of becoming injured.

Warm-up wonders

You may be surprised to know that you don't have to undertake a complex regimen of boring exercises to reduce your injury risk. Physiotherapists and researchers have come up with evidence-based programmes that work on women's weak spots, which, if performed for ten minutes, three times a week, can result in a 45% reduction in injury risk at the knee, and nearly a 30% reduction in overall injury risk.[23] They're called multi-component conditioning programmes[24] and they address muscle imbalance, muscle weakness and neuromuscular coordination in one hit.[25] It sounds complex, but it's simply a set of conditioning exercises that make us move in ways that stretch and strengthen muscles and make our brains work at using the right muscles at the right time. The best thing about them is that they don't take hours to do – in fact most are about ten minutes long – and can be incorporated into your warm-up or your existing programme as little as three times a week.

Help is at hand

You don't have to go it alone when it comes to including some really effective exercises into your workout to help build resilience to injury. If you google 'ACL injury prevention exercises' you'll find many links[26] and YouTube videos[27] giving some great examples of exercises you can do a few times a week that will make you more resilient to injury. These exercises won't just help you work out, they'll help you safely perform your daily activities. We're constantly bending, lifting and supporting children or elderly parents, hoovering, running around after dogs or children, doing DIY or moving furniture. Incorporating conditioning exercises into your life will help you move your body well, strengthen your muscles and create a strong, stable, mobile base from which to do all these activities, regardless of how much sport and exercise you do.

Warm up well

Here are some examples of the type of exercises you can include in your warm-up two or three times a week, or do as stand-alone fifteen-minute workouts, to help prevent injury during your swim, your run, your YouTube workout or your sports training sessions – but bear in mind that these exercises are not a substitute for the strength training that we also advocate. Once you're happy doing our top ten injury-prevention exercises below, mix in a few different variations or progressions.

And don't be tempted to skip these exercises just because you do similar ones in your HIIT or CrossFit workouts. The focus here is on technique, control and quality of movement – the very things that usually get thrown out the window when Barry is roaring at you to do five more jump squats in the last ten seconds of your bootcamp circuit. It's ten to fifteen minutes of intentional self-preservation a few times a week. Give yourself that gift.

Injury-resilience-building warm-up!

This warm-up is designed to help build strong, resilient girls and women who have great technique and movement patterns. It should take less than fifteen minutes, once you learn the exercises. You can see how-to photos at www.TheWell-HQ.com/warmup.

Basic guidelines

- Always focus on your technique.
- If possible, do the exercises in bare feet.
- Start slowly, and layer on strength and power once the technique is established.

Each exercise is to be done for one minute, slowly, intentionally, focusing on technique, rather than fitting as many in as you can.

- **Squat**
  1. Starting with your feet in line with your shoulders, move your hips back first, as if sitting down in a chair, keeping your weight evenly distributed over the whole foot.
  2. Remain slow and controlled on the way down, making sure the knees don't drop inwards.
  3. Push through the whole foot as you stand up.
  4. Advanced: Add a small jump at the start of your squat with a soft landing, focusing on landing mechanics (no knees knocking or caving in).

- **Split squat (one minute each leg)**
  1. Place one foot 50–80cm in front of the other, then raise the heel of your back foot.
  2. Drop down into a squat, looking ahead and keeping your torso long.
  3. Control the movement on the way down, keeping your knee in line with your foot.
  4. Drive up through the front foot.
  5. Advanced: Add a forward lunge, where you step forward and then back, alternating the leg you step forward on.

- **Hip hinge**
    1. Place your feet shoulder-width apart and slightly bend your knees, making sure your weight is going through the whole of each foot.
    2. Push your hips back while keeping the torso long.
    3. Your hip drives the movement, so your upper body will move because your hips are moving. As soon as the hips stop, the torso stops.
    4. Starting with the hips, drive back up.
    5. Advanced: Hold a single dumbbell or a kettlebell in both hands just beneath your belly button, between your hips; perform the hip hinge and power through the resistance provided by the weight.

- **Forward lunge**
    1. Walk forward into a lunge position – focus on knee alignment: your knee should be over your foot.
    2. Keep the torso long throughout.
    3. Advanced: Add an upper-body rotation either away, from or towards the front knee, as you step into the lunge.

- **Clock lunge**
    1. Imagining you're the middle of a clock, step forward with one leg to 12 o'clock and back to the centre.
    2. Work your way around the whole clock face – 12, 1, 2, 3, etc. – always keeping the body facing forward.
    3. On each lunge forward, step as far out of range as you can.
    4. Advanced: Reach forward with your arms, perhaps holding 1kg or 2kg weights, or a tin of tomatoes, in each hand, as you step forward.

- **Bridge**
    1. Lie on your back, feet flat on the floor.
    2. As you exhale, lift your hips off the floor and hold them up – keep your knees aligned over your feet and don't let them drop in or out.
    3. Build towards holding for one minute, breathing throughout – don't hold your breath.
    4. Advanced: Single-leg bridges – as above but with one leg outstretched.

- **Bird dog**
    1. On all fours, evenly distribute your weight through each knee and hand.
    2. On an exhale, extend opposite hand and foot, reaching as far back and forward as you can, slowly and with intention.
    3. Keep your weight evenly distributed on the remaining hand and knee, so you don't shift over to one side – this is really tricky to do well.
    4. After holding out the extended hand and foot for a couple of seconds, return to centre with control (no wobbling), then switch to the other hand and foot.
    5. Advanced: Hold the positions for longer and focus on keeping your core clenched.

- **Vertical jump**
    1. Starting with your feet shoulder-width apart, come down into a squat, then drive up as hard as you can and jump high.
    2. Land lightly and concentrate on your knees – they should be aligned with your feet, not dropping inwards.
    3. Add more power as your technique improves.
    4. Advanced: Jump off two feet and land on one.

- **Skip**
  1. Start with basic skipping – use a rope if you have one, otherwise imagining using one will do! – and focus on landing lightly to improve your body control.
  2. Add in power so that you're driving up through the knee and still landing lightly.
  3. Advanced: Move around the space in different directions.

- **Balance**
  1. Balance on one foot for 10–30 seconds at a time.
  2. Advanced: Make it more challenging by closing your eyes or by standing on an uneven surface then throwing and catching a ball or lifting your arms above your head. You should be wobbling, but not falling over.

Emma

Unlike Baz, who has a love of Olympic lifting and strength work (a hangover from her rowing days), I have always been very 'conditioning averse'. I like running, so I want to run. The trouble is, I am a walking advert for why that's a rubbish idea for staying injury-free, because ever since I took up running in my early twenties I have been hampered by joint injury in my back, hips, knees and ankles. The problem here wasn't that I didn't know about the benefits of conditioning work, nor that numerous physios hadn't given me great exercise programmes to try to fix my ailments. It was that I found the exercises they gave me boring; I made the excuse that I didn't have time for them, and that if I had forty-five minutes to work out in, I would much rather spend it running than dedicate a third of it to some boring conditioning regime. Except then I couldn't, because my injuries meant I was unable to run. That maths didn't add up! It was a false economy, because in the end I spent much less time running, instead nursing niggles and injuries, than the thirty minutes I would have lost each week fitting in some vital conditioning that might have prevented those niggles altogether!

Change your behaviour with a COM-B over

We know Emma's story isn't unique. We see the same pattern in others, ranging from Olympic athletes to fellow active women, and it poses a big problem: how do we get good habits to stick when it comes to ensuring we protect ourselves from this increased injury risk – or from anything else that puts our health and well-being at risk?

The three of us really like to use the 'COM-B' model of behaviour change to build in conditioning and injury-prevention exercises into your routine.[28]

The acronym COM-B stands for:

- **C is for Capability**

  Do you have the capability to do what you need to do? Do you understand exactly what it is you need to do and have instructions, examples, pictures or an instructor showing you what to do? Are you physically able to do the exercise with the right technique? Do you know what the right technique feels like? Can you watch yourself performing the movement to check? If you don't start at the appropriate level to give yourself a chance of achieving what you set out to do, you'll always feel like you're failing and won't be inclined to keep it up.

- **O is for Opportunity**

  Do you have the opportunity to incorporate these conditioning exercises into your week? Do you have the physical space, the equipment and the time? Can you improve your opportunity to include them by building them into something that you already like doing, such as a warm-up to your main sport, or organize a social opportunity by doing them in a group setting or finding an accountability buddy who'll do them with you or check with you that you've done them?

- **M is for Motivation**

  Do you know *why* you need to do this, and does that reason energize you enough to get you moving? Do you need more information to convince you? Do you need to think of the bigger picture, rather than just the short-term goal?

- **B is for Behaviour**

  If you can tick off all of these things, you're much more likely to actually adopt the behaviour of incorporating conditioning exercises (or any health habit you are trying to start) into your week, which will help you achieve your health and fitness goals.

Emma's sticking point was the 'M' – she wasn't motivated to do the exercises because she found them boring. And however much concentration even the easiest conditioning exercises required, they weren't challenging enough for her. Plus, they were infinite, without a clear start and end goal, which Emma found unrewarding. So, she tuned in to what motivates her: taking on a challenge. She began signing up for thirty-day challenges, all of them free and online, ranging from a thirty-day yoga challenge to a thirty-day handstand challenge. Each of the challenges included elements of the injury-prevention exercises, just in different guises. What really overcame Emma's motivation issues was reframing them, changing from thinking of them as pre-habilitation exercises into something more fun and that had a start and a finish, and a sense of accomplishment.

I am strong, I am invincible, I am woman

We realize that many women don't think that strength training and weights are for them. In fact, only 25% of women do any strength training at all.[29] Often, they don't want to add bulk to their bodies. But strength training rarely adds bulk unless you're following a designed-for-bulk programme and you work hard on your nutrition to support muscle growth. Most women won't gain bulk by accident; you have to be truly committed to doing so, and if you want to, you can.

Strength training supports the health of our muscles and bones, and gives us a fit, capable body. It is vital to a woman's ability to move well and stay injury-resistant, and to protecting her long-term health and well-being. A woman's physiology is actually not predisposed to make lots of new muscle, and as we age, our body is dead set on losing muscle, rather than gaining it. That's why strength training is so important across our whole life. We can be strong as women, and we can stay strong as we age – but that doesn't happen by itself!

Baz was lucky enough to have been taught from a young age how to lift weights, but this is not the case for most women. This is a problem because it means that many women don't have the confidence to step into the weights section of a gym, or we go in without a clue as to what to do and how to do it, and either injure ourselves or fail to make any progress. The barriers to women doing strength training are often not physical, but social. A 2021 survey of 400 women who were gym regulars found that 73% felt intimidated doing weights in the gym, and 64% felt safer exercising at home compared with a public gym due to being made to feel uncomfortable by men in the gym.[30] This gym culture is stopping women from doing weights despite the fact that, overall, there is a growing appetite in active woman to include weights in their training (the boutique gym chain Third Space says over 50% of those attending their strength-and-conditioning classes are women),[31] while online fitness communities led by women lifting weights and training for strength are hugely popular. What this tells us is that many women want to do strength training, but they don't feel confident or safe doing so. Changing this culture will take time, and will require a commitment from gyms and leisure centres, their users, trainers and the women who use them, to hold their ground and call out the bad stuff (so much easier said than done). But if it's confidence to use certain spaces in gyms that's putting you off, there are other ways to get your dose of strength training, whether that means going to some strength-training workout classes or following some of the brilliant online communities such as Alice Liveing, Jennis, @Doclyssfitness or @LauraBiceps.

Strength training works across our lives

Strength training is vital to anyone who loves training and competing but it's also key for all women at every life stage. Here's why:

- Developing a strong, resilient body is important as we hit puberty and our risk of joint injury starts to increase. Remember, we have a much greater risk of joint injury than men. Starting strength work and conditioning exercises from the moment we head into puberty and beyond really helps to create a body that is far less at risk of injury throughout our lives.
- We know that in girls with a healthy menstrual cycle, 90% of their bone density is laid down by the age of twenty, it peaks

by thirty, and from then on our bone strength is in a steady decline. But the great news is that strength training can slow this down and, in some cases, stop it in its tracks. As we're all living so much longer now, strength training really is a fundamental part of a woman's training routine to ensure we stay moving well to avoid injuries and falls through our midlife and later years.

- Strength training, done correctly, makes us better at other sports and hobbies. Baz worked with a group of midlife runners in Ireland who swapped out a couple of runs a week for weight training and they all reported running faster and having fewer niggles in terms of back pain and Achilles' heel problems. Even runners who were reluctant to change their approach at first saw the improvement in their running mates and shifted to prioritizing a couple of sessions a week to strength work.

- Weight training also helps us maintain our muscle mass as we age, which can help to slow down or stop weight gain in midlife. Cardio sessions are typically measured in calories burned; however, we know that the metabolic impact – the fat-burning potential – of a heavy weights session is far greater than a cardio session, and that muscle tissue you're making uses more calories at rest, even when your body isn't moving. As women's oestrogen levels start to fluctuate and drop in midlife, weight gain is a concern for many, and instead of doing more miles, having well-thought-out strength sessions in your fitness regime can help maintain body shape.

- The benefits of strength training are not just physical. Women who strength-train also report more positive feelings about their bodies than women who don't.[32] Strength training has also been shown to alleviate depression and to improve low mood and loss of interest in activities.[33]

Hopefully we've convinced you of the benefits of strength training. However, a lot of what we currently know about how to design strength-training programmes or workouts is – you guessed it – based on what has been shown to work to make men fitter and stronger. Our physiology is different, and we need plans and programmes that take this into account.

Getting on your nerves

Lots of people assume that with all their muscle-building testosterone, men respond much better to strength training and get stronger, quicker. In actual fact, with a well-planned programme, men and women make similar gains with strength training.[34] But what's pretty cool is that *how* we develop strength happens slightly differently. The way the body gets stronger isn't simply by making lots of new muscle. It's more sophisticated than that. The brain gets better at sending signals to the muscles to contract harder and in a more coordinated way, which produces more force. This is a universal adaptation when anyone starts doing strength work, but women go on to develop greater increases in strength through these nervous-system changes rather than continuing to build up more muscle tissue, as in men. It's a brain over brawn approach to getting strong, which doesn't result in bulky muscles.

What that means for women is that if we design our strength training to include lots of 'functional' movements – ones that use similar muscle patterns as the sports or activities we enjoy – then we can reap the benefits in better performance. We get strong by training our brains to talk to our muscles in a really efficient way. So, if you're a runner, including some strength work which uses the muscles in a running-specific way (like lunges and squats) will improve your running performance. How many times have you heard someone say they injured their back carrying heavy bags? Or tweaked their knee running for the train? Or put their hip out carrying a toddler having a tantrum? Training in this 'functional' way also improves your chances of avoiding a non-sport-related injury.

> ### Emma
>
> In my twenties, I researched the brain; more specifically, how well the brain sends signals to muscles under different conditions, like when we are too hot and have too little oxygen after marathons or strength training. True to the 'culture' of sports science research, I tested only males, or males and females together, giving no thought to the difference between sexes. At the time, I didn't question this approach, and I still feel slightly outraged at myself for not addressing the lack of attention then being paid to research in females. As if to right that wrong, years later, the first PhD student I ever supervised is now diligently working to understand the performance of females in his own research as an academic. He and his colleagues at Northumbria University are finding some interesting facts about how women's muscles get tired and produce less strength, which we've included in this chapter.[35]

Ain't no stopping us now

Far from being 'the weaker sex', women can actually outperform men when it comes to repeatedly performing strength exercises. Women are shown to be less susceptible to fatigue, which means that when they are doing strength exercises, they can go on for longer than men. And the difference isn't trivial: in research studies, women keep performing, rep after rep, for 60% longer than men doing the same resistance exercise.[36] Better still, in the second half of the menstrual cycle, when progesterone is high, this effect is amplified.[37]

So, how can you use this knowledge on the gym floor or in your workouts? You need to ensure that the last couple of reps you're doing in your sets are really tough (while still maintaining good technique). If you're not grinding out these last couple of reps, then you need to either increase the weight or up the reps, so that your muscles are really in a state of fatigue by the end of your set, otherwise they won't be stimulated enough to cause any adaptation, to get stronger and more powerful, and to reap all the rewards that come from that. If you're following a programme that has been designed on a male physiology, the number of reps that have been prescribed may not be enough to really get your female muscular system working!

What we get asked all the time about strength training

Every woman's goals for sport and exercise are different, and that influences what and how much strength training they choose to do. But whatever activity you choose to do, it should include strength training, for your health and lifelong mobility as much as for your enjoyment and success in sport and physical activity. Since strength training might be one of the last bastions of the male-dominated sports arena, women feel not only that they can't ask female-centric questions about strength work, but that the answers they'll get will probably still be fixed in the male-centric approach. That's what we, and this book, are here for.

FAQs

Here are some of the questions women ask us when they want to start or progress in strength training and our advice for getting it right.

Can women get stronger upper bodies?

In terms of absolute strength, women are, on average, about 50% less strong than men in their upper bodies (but only 30% less strong than men in their lower bodies).[38] But that doesn't mean we can't get strong there. In fact, research shows that when a group of women and men are subjected to the same upper-body strength training, women make better adaptations than men.[39] The researchers don't know exactly why, but it's likely because, on the whole, women do less upper-body training across their lives, and when you take someone who hasn't done training before and put them through a programme, you will usually find they respond better than others who are already well trained in those exercises. Not so much a case of beginner's luck as the big, initial changes in the brain, nervous system and muscles when you start learning something new. So, yes, women can get strong upper bodies, and because of the benefits of whole-body training on injury, mobility and daily functioning, we definitely should be training our upper body!

I train four times a week already. How am I going to find the time to add in extra sessions?

Many of us have established an exercise routine that works for us and our lives, so when you're considering starting strength training, think about how to incorporate it into your existing exercise schedule and don't just try to add more sessions in – inevitably these often get missed because you are short on time, energy or both.

I'm worried about leaking urine when I lift heavy weights. What should I do?

This is a fear and a reality for many women, and if you do experience any pelvic floor issues then help is available. Our recommendation is to train at a weight or rep range that doesn't give you symptoms and seek out the help of a women's health physio who understands that sport and training are important to you. They will be able to help you to incorporate your pelvic floor exercises into your training, which is the holistic approach we should all be working towards.

I'm on the pill. Will this affect my ability to gain strength?

It's unlikely, but if you're not seeing the gains you'd expect and you're training, fuelling and recovering well, then check that your pill is not one of the anti-androgenic ones, which have been shown to slow down women's strength gains.[40]

I have chronic lower back pain. Where do I start?

Don't give up on yourself. Movement is good for lower back pain, and pelvic floor work and strength training are often an important combination to help alleviate back pain. Physios can generally recommend trainers they trust or look for those qualified to work with your symptoms. Do your homework and make sure they have an approach you can work with – they need to treat you as a woman who has potential and neither like a fragile vase that's about to break nor someone who needs to ignore the pain and push through. These trainers should recognize your fitness level, teach you some fundamental movement patterns and set an appropriate programme. This may take anything from four to twelve sessions but will be a worthwhile investment of your time and money in the long run.

I just love doing my sport but I hate the gym. How can I do strength training?

Be creative and involve others. Is there a way that you can add some strength-and-conditioning work to your sport? It's really important, especially for those activities that are low-impact or non-weight-bearing, such as swimming or cycling, to make sure you are putting load through your muscles and bones with impact or weight. Because otherwise, regardless of how fit you are, your bone and muscle strength could still be in decline. To give you an idea, an eight-minute circuit including squats, lunges, burpees and skipping would be a great warm-up or finisher for cyclists, or swimmers could swap out one swim set in the pool for this type of HIIT session poolside.

Do I need to lift heavy weights or can I use a set of dumbbells?

If you're starting from scratch, then small dumbbells, resistance bands and bodyweight are all fine, but over time you will need to progress or your body won't change. The heavier we lift, the more of our muscles are used and the greater the effect on our muscles, bones and metabolism. But anything is better than nothing, so just get started with whatever feels right for you, knowing that you should aim to increase weights over time.

Can I lift weights with my children?

Yes, and it's a great way to get children who don't like running, catching or throwing to move and do exercise. The focus with children is always on technique, and if they learn how to move well as youngsters, it's a skill they'll never lose. Plus, it's a fun thing you can do together. But be aware of classes that use your children as weights! Babies are not weights and using them as such isn't good for your technique and leaves you prone to injury at a time that your body is more susceptible already, post-natally. There's a lot of equipment out there that you can use, so put the baby in the buggy or on a mat and have them watch you do your thing.

What are the best and the worst exercises?

This is one of our most popular but least favourite questions, as we really believe that there are no such things as good and bad exercises, just good and bad form. Having a good- and bad-exercise list is just not helpful. Having said that, Baz is obsessed with squats and feels that knowing how to squat well is as important as learning to read. Any movement that is fundamental to our lives is something that we should all know how to do. Go basic first, before getting fancy – and by basic we mean squat, deadlift, lunge, pull (rows, high-pull) and push (overhead press) movements. Add as much load to these as you can (always retaining great technique) and this will be a terrific place to start.

How many times a week should I lift weights, and for how long?

We recommend the following for a healthy woman of any age.

- Do six to eight different exercises.

- Do six to twelve reps of each exercise – remember to adjust the weight so the last couple of reps are really hard work.
- Change this up every six to eight weeks and increase the weight as the weeks progress.
- If you can only do weight-lifting twice a week, then try to add a couple of lifts into another session you do, or add in some bodyweight-conditioning at home.
- You'll need to do weights at least twice a week to see a difference – once a week won't lead to very much improvement.

I train with men and have a male coach. What should I be doing differently?

Don't throw the baby out with the bath water – not all training programmes are rubbish because they haven't been designed with a women's physiology in mind. Instead, try to approach your training in a more informed way and see how you can get the best out of your exercise.

I'm not getting any stronger. Why not?

If you're not making gains in strength and power, then go back to basics. Are you including enough progression to cause adaptation? This means that once a weight or number of reps feels easy, you need to increase the weight or do more reps. On the flip side, too much progression can cause inadequate recovery and potential over-training, which can stunt progress too. It's hard to get the balance right at first, so take a step back for a moment and look at your energy levels. If you feel like your energy is constantly flatlining, or that you're overwhelmed by everything, then it's likely that your body does not have the capacity to adapt to exercise. Your life circumstances can play a big part in this: your workload, who you care for, how you're managing stress and so on. All of these elements need to be considered when designing your training programme. Sometimes less is more and it may make you stronger, faster and healthier in the long run.

Do men and women need to do different exercises?

If you read the Sunday supplements, you'd think so – there are so many articles written where the men's exercises are described in terms of strength, power and force, and the women's pages generally include pictures of scantily clad women sitting down with pink dumbbells and exercises designed to tone, tighten or lift. Even the names of the workout classes have traditionally reflected this, from 'Bums 'n' Tums' to 'Sculpt and Tone'. Women need to lift weights, and to do it with great form. They may lift less weight than the men, but there are no 'girls-only' or 'just-for-men' movements – we should all be able to do them all.

Do I need to change my diet as well?

Active women need more protein to help their muscles repair and grow, and to perform other vital health and performance functions; meanwhile, well-timed carbs underpin energy, hormone health, performance and recovery. For many women, it's hard enough getting to the gym or training, let alone making sure that they're properly fuelled and hydrated before, during and after exercise. But this is key. Baz always says that we can train as hard we like but we have to make sure that the support is in place to make sure we're fully recovering from our exercise, and diet is an important part of this.

How to be a body that moves well

- Move in every way possible from a young age and don't limit your sporting activities to just one type, particularly as young women. Variety builds physical literacy and resilience.
- Proactively eliminate your increased injury risk as a woman. Add ten minutes of conditioning exercises into your routine three times a week and do them consistently.
- Check in with niggles and with your cycle by tracking. Do your menstrual hormones change how you move, or how movement feels? Adapt accordingly.
- Strength and conditioning should be a key part of any training programme, lifelong, for every woman. If you aren't sure how, or aren't confident in your technique, get help from a fitness professional, go to a group class or find good coaching online.

Chapter 8

Eating Well

Instead of 'bikini bodies' and 'weight-loss wonders', wouldn't it be amazing if food featured less in the context of what we looked like and more about how it makes us feel and function? What we eat is the foundation for good health and for physical and emotional well-being; it fuels movement and exercise, so it's a non-negotiable for great training and performance. What we eat can impact our health so much that an optimal diet can add ten years to our life expectancy.[1] Yet, despite being indispensable to our vitality, women generally have different attitudes towards food than men do. A research study of hundreds of male and female university students found that many more women had tried a low-fat or low-carb diet, and more women thought it was important to limit the amount of fats and carbohydrates they ate.[2] When asked about how our sex impacts what we eat, clinical nutritionist Yvonne Bishop-Weston suggests that women have more emotional attachments to food and, due to media pressure, they attach guilt to carbs and saturated fats, and often feel a responsibility to eat healthily, in ways that men don't.[3] But 'eating healthily' is a misleading expression: it's not healthy to consume fewer calories than you need. It's not healthy to cut out entire food groups like fats or carbs. It's not healthy to restrict or deprive yourself of food, striving to achieve a photoshopped body shape that's a fallacy of health.

A British rowing club has an Instagram account dedicated to the food that the male rowers eat, such is the impressiveness of the quantities often consumed. Rowers train hard, really hard, and those enormous meals are absolutely necessary, given the amount of energy expended across their training days. Yet, when we look at the eating behaviours of active women, there's less celebration of food, and more deprivation, restriction, not enjoying food and instead being hyper-aware of body size and shape. When it comes to the 'doing gap', the nutrition one is more of a chasm. All the advice in the world on what to eat and when to eat it is no good if a woman's emotional relationship with food is fundamentally flawed. Most of us know what's good for us to eat; most of us know what a healthy balanced diet should look like. It's just turning that knowing into doing that is really hard when it comes to the food we eat, because there's so much more tied up in our relationship with food than just knowing what's best.

In the 'google it' era of information, there's a distinct challenge around the 'knowing' part as well. How do we really know what's good for us when we're being sold so much baloney about supplements, potions and pills that are meant to be the golden bullets for our health and fitness? Nutrition, and in particular sports nutrition, is a big business. The global sports-nutrition market was valued at over $50 billion in 2018 and is expected to increase to over $81 billion by 2023.[4] Such a big commercial interest should always be a red flag when it comes to checking the science behind all the shiny tubs of powders and pills on the store shelf claiming to give you the health and performance prowess you've always dreamed of. Often you can get just as much benefit using a food-first approach – that is, making sure that your diet contains all the micro- and macronutrients you need, before you throw good money after bad in the supplement store on nutrients that come naturally and cost-effectively from fruit and veg at the greengrocers.

There's another big red flag with sports nutrition. Most of the nutritional advice and development of best practice in fuelling and supplementing sports performance has been conducted on men, with the results extrapolated for women.[5] Yet there is a growing body of evidence that shows that there are many differences between the nutritional needs of the sexes when exercising. For example:

- During exercise, women use more fats and fewer carbs to fuel their workout than men do, and during the second half of the menstrual cycle this fat-preferring, carb-sparing physiology is even more pronounced.[6] This means that a woman's body is better adapted to endurance or lower-intensity, steady exercise than high-intensity workouts. (That doesn't get you off the hook from doing both types of training; it's just our bodies are wired better for one type than the other.)
- The hormones of the menstrual cycle can influence the stability of our blood-sugar levels. In the second half of the cycle, there might be more peaks and crashes of blood sugar, which can affect our appetite and our mood.[7]
- A woman's window of opportunity to restock energy stores within her muscles, and help them repair following a workout, is shorter in women than men. You'll recover faster if you have a protein and carbohydrate snack within thirty minutes of finishing your exercise.[8]
- Women are at greater risk of not getting enough energy in their diet to support their active lifestyle and good health because they are more likely to overestimate the energy value of what they eat, restrict their food intake because of body dissatisfaction or societal pressures for a 'thin ideal', and/or have poor nutrition knowledge.[9]
- Active women are at an increased risk of iron deficiency. We lose iron during our periods, when we sweat and when we

do impact exercise, and we commonly don't eat enough food that's rich in iron.[10]

- Getting nutrition wrong, even unintentionally, can disrupt or completely knock out our menstrual cycle and its wonderful hormones, which has a knock-on effect on reproductive health, bone health, immune function, fitness and mental health.[11]

When you're an active woman, you can't expect to be at the top of your game for long if you're running on empty. You'll end up spluttering along, frustrated and exhausted. Women need to adopt good eating habits, including key nutrients, to support their active lifestyle and sports performance. Emma used to work with a sports nutritionist who coined the phrase 'unleash the power of food', and we always find that so empowering when it comes to how we think about what we eat. You have the opportunity to use food as a superpower, if you get it right.

Doing the basics brilliantly

We're going to start with the basics, because far from being simple and straightforward, they are the most powerful tool an active woman has in her armoury when it comes to eating for performance. Time and again, when we have treated, trained or coached women, we have seen, often unintentional, nutritional issues and the havoc this wreaks with health, well-being and fitness. Getting energy into your body in a way that suits female physiology and supports female hormone health can have widespread benefits. And it's not just your training that will benefit when you eat properly, it's all of your physiological systems. Failure to eat and drink the right amount means not only that your ability to be active becomes compromised, but that your ability to adapt to your training is affected. You can lose muscle mass rather than gaining it, your bone density can be weakened, your immune system can be compromised, you are more likely to be injured, and you can experience menstrual health dysfunction, to name just a few of the reasons why good nutrition is fundamental to thriving as an active woman.

Meet the mistress of fuels

Let's start with carbohydrates. On a reality-TV series beloved in the UK, the female cast of *The Only Way is Essex* would cry, 'No carbs before Marbs!' to describe their approach to eating before their holiday to Marbella. But contrary to being your enemy, when consumed in the right way carbohydrates – carbs – are quite literally your best friend when it comes to having a fit, healthy body. Carbs are often referred to by nutritionists as the 'master fuel' because they are the fuel the body can use whether it's doing short bursts of high-intensity exercise or lower-intensity, longer-duration exercise.[12]

Carbs fuel pretty much everything we do. Carbs are also the only energy source used by our nervous system (including our brains). When we're at work or school all day, carbohydrates are vital for our cognitive performance. Active women are really good at using fat as a fuel source but, even when we do, carbs still play an important part in that process, because the body uses them to break down fat to make energy. And if that wasn't enough, if we don't have enough carbs in our system when we're exercising, our body starts to break down the protein in our muscle, converting it to glucose to use as fuel. After exercise, muscles cannot repair well or get stronger if we don't replace our carbohydrates quickly.[13] We can literally reverse the effect of training if we don't have carbs to burn. Training should help *build* muscle, not *lose* it. Save muscle: eat carbs!

A woman's hormones are especially sensitive to carbohydrate levels. Remember how our menstrual cycle starts in our brain?

The hypothalamus and pituitary gland in our brain send signals down to our ovaries to start the release of oestrogen and progesterone across the cycle. This signalling pathway from the brain to the ovaries starts to malfunction if we don't have enough energy coming in from carbohydrates. If levels drop too low, the signal from our brain to our reproductive system starts to falter, and eventually stops, at which point our menstrual cycle disappears.

Research has shown that it's not just the total number of calories we eat that's important, but also the timing of that energy intake – keeping blood sugar stable and not having long periods where our body is deprived of energy. One study proved that it wasn't a woman's bodyweight or the overall number of calories she consumed in a given day that put her most at risk of interrupting her hormone signals; rather, it was going through long periods with low energy – either by not eating at regular intervals, being active without having eaten beforehand or not replenishing energy after being active – that led to the disruption in the menstrual cycle.[14]

How often and when should I ideally eat?

As an active woman, to keep your body and your reproductive hormones happy and healthy you should aim to eat at least every three hours. Eat or drink a snack or meal containing carbs before you train – yes, even if that training is first thing in the morning and you have to get up twenty minutes earlier to munch on something – it doesn't have to be a full-blown brekkie, either; just a banana or a cereal bar to boost your energy levels for your session. After exercise, have a carbohydrate-and-protein snack within about thirty minutes of finishing. This is the peak time for women's bodies to refuel and repair their muscles.

Women are really bad at eating to fuel their sporting activities with research consistently showing that active women don't typically eat enough carbohydrates to compensate for their energy expenditure.[15] Whether it's women exercising to stay healthy, or elite athletes training to perform at the highest level, we are simply not eating enough carbs. Take the England women's national football team. This is a team of athletes with two nutritionists and a performance chef working to support them. Yet when those nutritionists, led by Dr James Morehen, conducted a study to see whether the squad were eating appropriately to meet the demands of their training camp and matches, they found that only one player out of the squad of twenty-four consumed enough carbs in their diet.[16] And 88% of the players didn't eat enough calories to match what they were expending every day. It's easy to think that if you can't get it right with a nutritionist and a performance chef at your disposal, what's the point? But there are some simple steps we can take to help us hit our carb targets.

At the most basic level, we need to ensure that at least half of what we put on our plates at each meal, or eat in snacks, is carbs. If you want to work out more specifically how much *you* need, multiply your bodyweight in kilograms by six, and that will give you your daily carb requirement in grams. So, a 65kg active woman needs 6 x 65 or about 390g of carbs each day.[17] As a guide, you'll get 50g of carbs from either two thick slices of wholewheat brown bread, a medium baked potato, a bowl of wholewheat spaghetti (65g dried), two bananas, a plain bagel or an 80g bowl of porridge. To ensure your diet includes the optimum mix of essential nutrients:

- include carbs like wholegrains, fruit and vegetables, as these are also full of fibre, which is vital for gut health and for vitamins and minerals, which are proven to support health and prevent disease
- choose complex carbs like brown bread or rice, sweet potatoes, beans and lentils
- skip the simple sugars; although sugar is a carbohydrate,

eating foods high in sugar such as cakes, pastries, sweets and sugary drinks is not the way to get your carbs in – sugar wreaks havoc with energy levels, and is shown to be bad for long-term health

There are apps that enable you to check the carbohydrate, protein and fat intake in your daily diet. But beware of using food tracking apps every day, because this can become an obsession. If you're worried about your diet, or wondering whether it stacks up, use a diet-tracking app for just a couple of days when you feel like your eating is normal for you and have a look at your diet's energy value (total calories) and macronutrient breakdown (how much carbohydrate, protein and fat you eat). This will give you a good idea of what your overall diet looks like, and the women we work with are often surprised by what it shows them, compared with what they thought their diet consisted of!

Emma

I worked with a teenage female triathlete who came to me because she was struggling with her energy levels, her periods had stopped five months previously and she had been performing poorly at races. In an otherwise healthy teenager, whose blood tests came back all clear from her doctor, the signs pointed to her diet being the source of the problems. However, she was convinced that she was eating really well: she was a healthy bodyweight for her height and age, her diet was varied, she had regular meals, lots of veg, and also enjoyed cake and biscuits. She was puzzled by how she could be getting her nutrition wrong when she thought she was careful about fuelling her high training-load well. We used a food-logging app to look at what she was eating and when she was eating it, alongside her training diary. She carefully monitored training and diet for a week, which shouldn't be underestimated as a task, because it takes some commitment, but it was very revealing.

Even though she was eating an excellent, balanced diet, there were three main flaws. When we looked at the energy that her training required, we found that her diet was consistently coming up short – some days by not much, other days by about 500 calories. She also wasn't eating enough carbohydrates. And finally, she was terrible at pre- or post-exercise fuelling, sometimes skipping breakfast before an early training session, leaving it ninety minutes after training before having anything to eat or having one piece of fruit to tide her over until her next main meal, hours later. But small adjustments in these three areas meant that within three months her periods returned. She also reported a PB, something she had been chasing for the previous six months. By helping this athlete to get the basics right for her female physiology, we made a complete U-turn from going down a road that could have had a negative impact on this athlete's health and performance, now and in the future.

Load me up

If you're into endurance sports, then you've no doubt heard of carb-loading. It's a practice where you ensure that, as well as tapering your training in the days before a big event – a marathon, an Olympic-distance triathlon, a long hike or a multi-game netball tournament – you fill your muscles to the brim with carbohydrates. Your bowls of pasta and piles of potatoes get stored in your muscle as glycogen and are used as fuel during exercise. This practice is based on research that shows a connection between how well we can maintain a given pace throughout endurance exercise and how much muscle glycogen we have at the start.[18] Carb-loading has shown benefits in exercise lasting more than ninety minutes. Starting your event – whether it's a football match or a marathon – with enough carbohydrates means that you can go longer (or faster) before hitting the dreaded 'wall' – the point where you have no more carbs left to fuel your movement and you grind to what feels like a halt.

And there's a big difference between the sexes when it comes to carb-loading. A study of athletes practising carb-loading before a performance test showed that in men who carb-loaded, stores of muscle glycogen increased by 40% and this translated into a 45% improvement in endurance performance.[19] In women, following the same carb-loading regime, no increase in muscle glycogen stores and no improvement in performance was observed.

This research group dug deeper to find out more about the sex difference. They found that during carb-loading where the instructions were to eat 75% of your daily calories as carbo-hydrates, since men generally eat more overall than women, their carb intake was proportionally greater.[20] In practice, then, carb-loading for women is really hard because to match the men, they'd need to eat more to get that performance-enhancing effect, which would in reality likely lead to weight gain rather than better racing.

If you're eating a well-balanced diet with enough carbs, com-bined with the taper – a big reduction in training – the week before a race or event, you'll likely be getting enough carbs to cross the starting line fully-fuelled. But if you want to be sure, increase your carb intake slightly – from 6g to 8g per kg of body-weight, to be specific – in the three to five days before your big event, and eat more calories overall from all the food groups on these days too. You might shift from 2,500kcals a day with 60% from carbs to 3,250kcals with 70% from carbs for the days leading up to your race.

Another important part of your nutrition preparation is to

make sure you make a good fuelling plan to keep your carbs topped up during the event. This in-event nutrition should be real food, if possible, rather than energy gels (it's absorbed better, to give you a steady and bigger supply of energy). Think brownie bites, bite-size sandwich portions with peanut butter and jelly, banana bread, dates and flapjacks. Make sure you practise with these foods during exercise in the lead-up to your big event. Exercise and eating are a notorious combination for causing gastrointestinal distress – typically bloating, nausea, pain and discomfort – so make sure you know what works for you to keep your energy levels topped up and your tummy feeling good for your big, long events.

Protein packs a punch

While carbohydrate gets the title of 'mistress of fuels', protein can take the 'supernutrient' crown. Protein plays an important role in virtually all body processes, including immune function, hormone health, and tissue repair and growth. If you want to stay fit and healthy, and adapt your training to grow fitter and stronger, then protein should be an important component of your diet.

For average women (by which we mean those who exercise three to five times a week, work, and have other responsibilities), it's easy to miss out on protein, especially if you tend to grab-and-go with snacks and meals. You can easily reach the end of the day having existed mostly on carbs: cereal for breakfast, a hummus-and-veggie bagel or a pasta pesto snack box for lunch. It can be hard to include protein in the mix, yet active women should aim to make protein 25–35% of their calorie intake.[21] Think of that as at least a quarter of whatever you put on your plate. What's important to note about protein is that the body has a limited ability to store it, so there's no advantage to having lots in one sitting, then none throughout the rest of the day.

Unlike carbs, you can't 'load' protein. The good news is that research shows that if active women get roughly the right amount of calories overall in their day, they are generally eating enough protein in the process.[22] However, athletes who are aiming for a particular bodyweight (often a lighter one) have been shown to be at risk of not getting enough protein.

If you're training more than three times a week, including certain proteins in a pre-training meal or snack can help your performance. The essential amino acids leucine, isoleucine and valine are different from other proteins as they are readily available energy sources for the body, and so these are good to include in a pre-training snack. These amino acids are found in meat – particularly poultry and beef – fish, eggs, chickpeas, nuts, seeds and brown rice. Including protein in your pre-exercise meal also slows down the depletion of your body's carbs, fends off fatigue, and can also help delay mental fatigue, which occurs as we get more physically tired during exercise.[23]

For very active women (those exercising more than five times a week), the overall protein requirements are greater than for those who don't exercise at all, and the need is greatest during recovery from exercise. Although we've said you need to consistently get protein hits throughout the day, research shows that it's your post-exercise protein that is essential for your recovery, for maintaining or improving your muscle mass, and for promoting optimal health.[24] So, pretty important then! Muscles have to repair and get stronger after training no matter what type of exercise we do and what type of fitness goals we're pursuing. The key here is to take advantage of the window of opportunity straight after your workout. After your training, your body is geared up to help your muscles repair and grow, so to take advantage of this, eat some protein within thirty minutes of finishing your training that is high in essential amino acids, such as quinoa, eggs, cottage cheese, turkey or fish. Not only will that support your adaptation to training, it can also improve your immune function – which can be compromised in this window following exercise – and reduce that post-workout muscle soreness.

Once again, women and men don't have exactly the same response to post-exercise eating: research suggests women need more protein than men after exercising to achieve maximum benefits.[25] There are endless options for your post-workout snack or meal that fit the carbohydrate and protein dose you require, and you don't have to over-engineer it – simple is good! A food-first approach that aims to supply all you need from your diet, before adding supplements, is the best way to get your nutrients. But if you're struggling to get enough of the right type of protein, then whey-protein powder mixed into milk or smoothies can also help. Below are some of our favourite post-exercise snacks.

 Our favourite recovery snacks

Grab-and-go:
- peanut butter and jam on a bagel
- Greek yoghurt, tahini, maple syrup and pumpkin seeds
- a smoothie of whizzed-up banana, almond milk and two scoops of whey protein
- pot of left-over pasta and pesto with peas

Cook it up:
- sweet potato topped with beef chilli or tuna mayo and sweetcorn
- beans on toast topped with feta or cheddar cheese
- egg fried rice with peas, ham and mushroom
- smoked salmon, scrambled egg and spinach in a pita-bread pocket – sprinkle on chilli flakes for heat

In-exercise fuelling

We've talked about making sure you have a pre-exercise meal, and that you seize the post-exercise window of opportunity for refuelling, but what about during exercise itself? There are so many in-exercise fuelling solutions on the shelves of running and cycling stores these days, from gels to chews, but again, this is where simpler is often better. The first rule of thumb when it comes to in-exercise nutrition for endurance events is 'drink to thirst, fuel to plan'.

Drink to thirst

Thirst is a good indicator of hydration. If you drink when you're thirsty, you're likely to stay hydrated, which is key when you exercise. Blood is largely made up of water, and the more hydrated you are, the greater your blood volume. This is important because blood transports energy to working muscles and takes the waste away. As well as staving off fatigue by delivering the energy to muscles, blood also helps us stay cool during exercise. That's why dehydration of as little as 2% of your body mass can lead to impaired performance. Plain water works fine for training sessions lasting up to about an hour, but if you're doing longer training or you're training in hot climates, you may benefit from the addition of electrolytes to your drink. You can do this by adding a dissolvable electrolyte tablet or by adding freshly cut or crushed fruit and herbs to your water bottle to create your own flavoured, electrolyte-infused water. Coconut water is also a great electrolyte-rich drink.

Fuel to plan

Unlike thirst, hunger is a signal that happens way too late for us to get the timing of fuelling right if we haven't planned for our body's energy needs, especially when we're exercising. It's a balance between getting energy in to top up your stores of carbohydrates when they become depleted, but not eating too much or fuelling with carbohydrate that is so concentrated it causes a stomach upset. In her Ironman triathlon, Emma spent the first half of the race fuelled with real food – jam sandwiches and fruit loaf – which worked well, keeping her fuelled without causing her gastrointestinal distress. In the second half of the marathon leg, she resorted to quick-fix gels, which proved to be too concentrated a form of sugar for her stomach to handle. What happens when you have such a rich dose of carbohydrates in something like a gel is that it's so concentrated your body actually has to draw water into your stomach to dilute it down, before it can send it around the body as energy. Drawing water into your stomach dehydrates you, and causes bloating, diarrhoea and stomach pain. This is exactly what Emma endured for the last ten miles of her Ironman – thank goodness for portable toilets!

The 'fuel to plan' strategy is to practise your in-exercise eating and drinking before you get to your big race. Emma used single gels quite consistently during long runs in training without experiencing any issues, but ten hours into the race, her body was working really hard to find energy, fend off fatigue and stay hydrated; what it really needed was something that was easy to digest and kind on the stomach, which the gels were not. As much as gels seem easy and convenient, the next time Emma embarked on something that long – a 100km ultra-endurance foot race in the South Downs in Sussex – she stuck to real food all the way. Despite being on her feet for over twelve hours, there wasn't a stomach cramp or an emergency pit-stop in sight!

Eating fats doesn't mean being fat

Just as carbs and protein are worthy of their own section in this chapter, fats, too, deserve recognition, not only because they are an important fuel source, but also because, especially in women, they are vital for cell health throughout our body, they help us absorb certain vitamins and they make sure our hormone levels stay balanced and healthy.

Despite the importance of getting enough fat in our diets, active women are the worst culprits for restricting their fat intake, believing that eating fat equals *being* fat.[26] It is recommended that active women consume at least 20% of their energy intake as fats, because women burn fats more during exercise than men do – we are brilliant fat-burning machines during low-intensity exercise![27] Research shows that when fat intake falls below this level, the muscle's fat stores are depleted after exercise and you can't perform as well in your next workout.[28] Since fats provide more than twice the energy per gram of protein or carbs, they are a very important and effective way for active women to get enough energy. There are right and wrong kinds of fats to include in your diet, however.

Which types of fat should you eat?

Not all fats are alike so it's important to have a healthy balance of fat types. Your diet should include foods with natural sources of saturated fats, such as meat – including poultry, beef and pork – and whole-fat dairy products. You may have heard that saturated fats are the bad guys, but actually it's when food is highly processed that saturated fats are the problem – fast food, fried products, sugary baked goods and processed meats are likely to affect health differently from a diet that contains modest amounts of saturated fats in the form of full-fat dairy and grass-fed meats. A healthy diet should also include monounsaturated and polyunsaturated fats, found in seeds, nuts, oily fish (salmon and trout), flaxseed oil, olive oil and avocados. It's also essential to incorporate foods rich in omega-3 and omega-6, such as flaxseeds, soybeans, oily fish and walnuts. As well as being beneficial to your general health, these fats have positive anti-inflammatory effects, which can reduce muscle pain and accelerate recovery – ideal factors for active women.[29]

High-fat diets

A high-fat, low-carb diet is often known as a ketogenic, or 'keto', diet. The low level of carbs in the diet causes your body to use fat as its main fuel, and when it burns fats, it makes things called ketones. The diet claims that you have to be in ketosis for your body to burn fat at a higher rate, which is why some people choose this method to diet. However, this is not an entirely accurate claim since you can be burning fat brilliantly and not produce ketones if there is adequate carbohydrate and protein in your diet. There have also been studies that show that this sort of diet is not optimal for active women because they need a balance of carbohydrates and fats to fuel different intensities of exercise.[30] Research shows that active individuals following high-fat, low-carb diet regimes perform poorly in high intensity exercise which relies on carbohydrate for energy production. In one study, peak power was reduced by 7% and distance covered during an intermittent sprinting test was down by 15% after just four days of a low-carbohydrate, ketogenic diet.[31]

Low-fat diets

In low-fat versions of foods, the fat that the manufacturer removes is often replaced with carbs such as starch and sugar, or worse, synthetic forms of sugar. In addition, when we remove fats from our diet by eating low-fat foods, we lose the very nutrient that is so important for energy, hormone health and immune function. Not only do we miss out on the essential function of fat in the diet, but low-fat foods are also unsatiating. They simply don't fill you up, yet they cause your blood sugar to spike, and unstable blood sugar can lead to food cravings, poor concentration and mood swings. The irony is that this spike in blood sugar causes insulin to be released, and this peak of insulin can cause a surge in cortisol – and this particular combination of hormones actually tells your body to store fat.[32]

Spotlight on fasted training

Fasting has become very popular in the past decade. It's promoted as a 'well-being' practice, with fasting retreats and plenty of celebrity endorsement for different fasting regimes. Fasting refers to restricting food – not eating – for certain periods of time. Intermittent fasting, for example, suggests people go for periods of between sixteen and twenty-four hours without eating. These recommendations are based on the fact that humans, as hunter-gatherers, are well equipped to go for some time without food, because for our ancient ancestors a hunt wasn't always successful, meaning food wasn't always immediately available, and nor were food preservation techniques yet invented as a way to make the supply of food more consistent.

However, there is still no robust evidence-base underpinning the health benefits of fasting in non-obese individuals, and the practice of training while fasting really goes against the needs of female physiology.[33] Indeed, research has shown that men respond better to fasted training, which emphasizes the need to look at nutrition for active women with a female filter applied. A key way to stay healthy, happy and fulfil your performance potential is to eat enough to fuel your training and your life. Fasting doesn't help you do that.

Fasted training gathered interest well before intermittent fasting was all the rage. Consciously opting to do fasted training – either not eating before you train or exercising while following an intermittent fasting diet – are all roads that lead you to work out in a fasted state. The practice of fasted training became a popular tool for coaches and athletes because of its potential to improve adaptation to endurance training. Research showed that if we trained in a fasted state, we started to more quickly use our fat stores as a fuel source (as opposed to using carbs), and when study participants consistently trained in a fasted state for six weeks, the endurance improvements that naturally come with training were amplified, compared with a group who ate before their workout.[34] This was an exciting prospect for all athletes: by not eating before they trained, they could get more bang for their buck when it came to fitness gains. Getting fitter, faster, is everyone's dream, right?

However, if it seems too good to be true, then it probably is. This early research has been superseded by studies that show the effects of fasted training are not all positive. One investigation has since found that running in a fasted state yields twice the amount of muscle breakdown than in a non-fasted state, which can actually decrease muscle mass and strength over time.[35] A meta-analysis of fasted training found that people were able to perform endurance exercise for longer after eating compared with when they fasted, so performance benefitted from a pre-exercise meal.[36] Fasted training also has a negative impact on how much and hard you can train. This makes sense because as we increase the intensity of our session, we have to use carbohydrates as fuel – it's the quickest way to make energy. And if we don't have carbs to pull energy from, the intensity of our workout is going to suffer.[37]

But women's bodies are already excellent at burning fat during exercise, so one of the benefits of fasted training – using more fats as fuel – we've already got nailed. For active women, the risks of fasted training go beyond not getting as much out of your training session or having a negative effect on muscle adaptation. The impact can be far more serious. Importantly, fasted training creates a state of low energy availability. Think back to our earlier discussion about how important it is to have a consistent energy source available, particularly carbohydrates, for the health of our hormone signalling and, consequently, of our menstrual cycle. Research shows that periods of low energy availability, such as during fasted training, are enough to cause menstrual dysfunction, by interrupting the release of your menstrual cycle hormones.[38] This has significant consequences for your overall health and your ability to train and perform at your best.

In women, one of the knock-on effects of fasting is that the concentration of the stress hormone cortisol increases. Having chronically elevated levels of cortisol, which can happen if you repeatedly train while fasting, can have a negative impact on reproductive hormones, as well as your overall health and well-being.[39] Baz has seen this on plenty of occasions in women who are keen to lose weight because of their changing physiology and body shape during perimenopause when their bodies start their natural transition to menopause. They often eat less or turn to fasting regimes, which sends the body into a 'fight or flight' cortisol response, which in turn stimulates fat storage, so you end up gaining, rather than losing, weight. The key to maintaining a healthy weight is to stabilize your blood sugar and keep cortisol in check by eating regularly.

So it's a no from us on fasted training. That's not to say that female athletes should never train without having eaten beforehand – sometimes logistics just work out that way. It's just not a good idea to make a habit of it, and particularly not a good idea to do high-intensity or long (more than ninety minutes) sessions without fuelling well before and afterwards. If someone told you to follow a regime that made your training less effective, gave you fewer fitness gains and put you at risk of getting ill or injured, you'd ignore that advice. But by doing fasted training (or by following a fasting regime while leading an active lifestyle), that's the choice you're making.

Putting our diet under the microscope

Micronutrients, which we often refer to as vitamins and minerals, are an important consideration in our diet. As their name suggests, we only need small quantities of these, but if we don't get the recommended amount, it can have significant consequences for our health, well-being and performance. Because micronutrients are not produced in our body, with the exception of vitamin D – which, in addition to getting from food, our bodies make when our skin is exposed to sunlight – we must get them from our diet, and in active women it's not uncommon to get the balance slightly wrong. When it comes to women's health, there are a few micronutrients that we'd like to look at in detail.

Pumping iron

Women risk iron deficiency because we lose iron in our menstrual blood, and active women are even more at risk because high-impact exercise causes red blood cells to rupture and die.[40] We also lose iron through urine and sweat. Our higher demand means that active women often don't meet their iron intake needs through their diets; it has been estimated that as many as 60% of exercising women have an iron deficiency.[41]

We get iron in our diet through two sources – haem and non-haem. Haem iron is more easily absorbed by the body and is found only in animal foods such as beef, fish and poultry. Non-haem iron is found in plant-based foods such as soya, dried fruit, legumes, fortified cereals, green leafy veg and wholegrains. To help your body absorb the iron in these plant-based foods, eat them alongside foods which are high in vitamin C, or with foods that contain haem iron.[42]

Taking iron supplements when you don't need them has its

own troublesome side effects on your gastrointestinal and cardiovascular systems, so don't just guess that your iron is low; ask your doctor to give you a blood test for iron if you suspect you might be deficient – the symptoms include fatigue, light-headedness and lethargy.[43] Bear in mind that reversing iron deficiency can take up to six months.

Bony C and Sunny D

The micronutrient calcium is the CEO of bone health: it builds, repairs and maintains our bones – which is vital for active women, who continually put demands on their bones to be strong and healthy – as well as being integral to blood clotting, fluid regulation and making sure our nerves can send signals throughout our body effectively. The reason vitamin D and calcium go hand-in-hand is that we can't absorb calcium without the help of vitamin D. So, when you're deficient in vitamin D, you're also doing your body out of the amazing effects of calcium. Research shows that women who restrict their diet, have disordered eating or actively avoid dairy products or other calcium-rich foods can also be susceptible to low calcium.[44]

Calcium and vitamin D also have some of the strongest evidence for being effective in reducing symptoms of premenstrual syndrome, or PMS. Vitamin D is actually a steroid hormone, and is essential for the health of our hormonal responses and for helping us ovulate, and research shows that women with diets rich in vitamin D and calcium are at lower risk of developing PMS.[45] These findings led researchers to look at using calcium- and vitamin-D-rich diets or supplements to improve PMS symptoms, and there is strong evidence to suggest that this is one of the most effective strategies in combatting PMS. Only a limited number of foods contain vitamin D, including fatty fish, fish liver oils, egg yolks, cheese and beef liver, so exposing the skin to sunlight is how we get 70–80% of the vitamin D our body needs.

Foods rich in calcium include milk, cheese and other dairy products, as well as fish where you can eat the bones, such as sardines, and green leafy veg.

Supplementing your diet with vitamin D is recommended during the winter months when there are fewer hours of daylight. You can ask your doctor for blood tests to check your calcium and vitamin D levels. If you are deficient, aim to increase their sources in your diet and, if necessary, consider taking supplements.

If you're thinking about using vitamin D or calcium supplements, here are some recommendations:

- Calcium citrate is easiest for the body to absorb and you don't have to take it with food.
- Calcium carbonate supplements are cheaper, but the body can't extract as much calcium from them and you need to take them with food for optimal absorption.
- Vitamin D is best absorbed into your bloodstream when paired with high-fat foods, so taking your supplement with a meal gives you a better chance of feeling the benefits.[46]

Magical magnesium

Magnesium is important for bone and cardiovascular health as well as for blood-pressure control, and it forms the basis of hundreds of reactions that happen in our body every second to keep it functioning well. It has a role in calming the nervous system and regulating the signals that are passed from your brain to the ovaries. It has also been shown to help keep oestrogen levels healthy and regulate our production of insulin, which keeps our blood sugar stable and helps our thyroid function correctly.[47] Having enough of the micronutrient magnesium helps everything from muscle cramps to insomnia.[48] When it comes to our menstrual cycle, the naturopathic doctor Lara Briden describes it as her first-line recommendation for healthy cycles, especially for women with polycystic ovary syndrome (PCOS), PMS or period pain.[49] Phew! That is a ton of responsibility for a small micronutrient! Yet it is often overlooked when we think about eating well.

If your diet contains lots of magnesium-rich foods, such as leafy green veg, wholegrains, legumes, nuts and seafood, and you manage stress effectively, you are probably getting enough magnesium. The body excretes more magnesium when we're stressed, however, which can lead to magnesium deficiency.[50] Although we can't easily test our magnesium levels, because most of it is stored inside our cells and so isn't detected in blood or urine tests, the symptoms associated with low magnesium can be muscle weakness, cramping, pins and needles, and irritability.[51] The best thing about increasing your magnesium intake through your diet, or supplements, is that you are likely to feel the results quite quickly.

Don't skimp on zinc

Like magnesium, zinc is important for many different functions in our body, including its role in our immune system, in making and transporting all kinds of hormones, and in turning our food into energy. It's particularly important for active women due to its role in muscle growth and repair, which make it essential in recovery from exercise. In fact, because athletes train, and recover from training, frequently, they have been found to have lower zinc levels, despite eating more than non-active people. This is because the body loves zinc to help it recover and adapt to training, so the more active you are, the more zinc you need.

Research has shown that zinc also plays a role in healthy ovulation and in alleviating period pain,[52] while zinc deficiency can lead to irregular periods and worsen your symptoms. Your body can't actually store zinc, so it needs a consistent supply, but if you're eating a diet that contains zinc-rich foods such as beef, fish, eggs, wholegrains, legumes and dairy, then you're unlikely to be deficient. You can have your zinc levels checked with a blood test.

Every November, UK Sport's doctors send Olympic and Paralympic athletes 'winter survival kits' to try to reduce the number of days' training they might lose to illness over the winter months.[53] Elite athletes are four times more likely to become ill in winter, particularly over the Christmas holiday season, due to a break from training, a slight relaxation of regular eating patterns, an increase in social events and, consequently, exposure to germs. This can then affect an athlete's training in January. As well as ordering a hold on all mistletoe, these survival kits contain instructions on good hand-washing (a simple yet effective way to stop the transmission of germs – as we all know so well, since Covid-19) and zinc lozenges. A recent research study suggests that zinc can help prevent upper respiratory tract infections and shorten the duration of viruses such as the common cold.[54] In the study, 75mg/day of elemental zinc taken in lozenges reduced the duration of upper respiratory tract infections by three days when taken less than twenty-four hours after the onset of symptoms and for the duration of the illness. The dose is important to note, as many over-the-counter lozenges contain too little zinc. Scientists believe that zinc acts as an antiviral agent and has antioxidant and anti-inflammatory properties that can help our immune system fight off viruses more quickly.[55]

Eating your way round the cycle

Since nutrition is such an important part of hormone health and improving your menstrual cycle experience, the three of us are often asked, 'Should I eat differently across my cycle?' Our philosophy is that nutrition works best when you take a consistent approach. Nutrition is as much about the 'doing' as the 'knowing' and making the 'doing' bit as simple and easy as possible is often the key to instilling healthy habits. Ensuring your diet includes enough magnesium or that you stay hydrated is much easier if this becomes part of your daily life, rather than you having to work out which day of the cycle you're on and what type of food might be best that day. Remembering to take your omega-3 supplement the day before your period starts is going to do very little to reduce your period pain; taking it consistently across weeks and months might possibly mean you have very little period pain at all.

That said, if you're finding that the day before your period is a low-energy time for you, your diet on those days might focus more on energizing foods. Or, if you find that caffeine makes your premenstrual headaches worse, you might opt to avoid it in the days leading up to your period. Or you might start taking advantage of your amazing energy and motivation in the first half of your cycle by training more – always remembering that more training means you'll need more protein and carbs to fuel your exercise and recovery. Rather than syncing diet with your cycle, apply what you know about *your* body and *your* cycle to use food in a way that helps.

Go with your gut

Gut health is having a moment, and it's about time, too. Our awareness of the importance of gut health has never been greater, and our understanding of the role the gut plays in our body's functioning is improving all the time. Your gut is home to trillions of microbes, which make up your gut microbiome, including bacteria, viruses and yeasts. This microbiome is known to interact with many other physiological systems, from our immune system to our hormone system and the neurophysiology in our brain. For example, recent research has shown that 80% of your immune cells live in your gut, where they help to ensure we have the right type of immune response to any threats, excrete antibodies and enhance our anti-inflammatory response.[56]

The gut–brain relationship is also being increasingly explored, with fascinating findings emerging about the role that the gut microbiome plays in anxiety and other mental health disorders. Researchers have found that they can use interventions that alter the gut microbiome to treat conditions such as anxiety.[57] What's interesting about these studies is that while supplementing with a probiotic can be an effective strategy, manipulating diet alone to improve the diversity of the microbiome (without the need to supplement) proved to be the better approach, with up to 86% effectiveness in reducing anxiety symptoms.

Among the numerous bacteria in the gut is a set called the estrobolome, which can influence the amount of oestrogen in our body. Now, we love to celebrate the power of awesome oestrogen, as long as it's balanced by progesterone. In excess, oestrogen can make our cycle symptoms worse, or even lead to more chronic conditions. When our gut microbiome is healthy and diverse, with a range of 'good' bacteria in there, our oestrogen levels remain healthy. When we have poor gut health – bad bacteria and a limited variety – our oestrogen levels can go haywire. The gut microbiome regulates oestrogen by releasing an enzyme called beta-glucuronidase, which 'reactivates' oestrogen that was on its way out (through our poo) and sends it back into circulation. Now, if this enzyme in the gut is too plentiful, instead of being excreted through your stools, too much oestrogen gets reactivated and sent back into the body, leading to an excess of oestrogen. By contrast, if not enough oestrogen is reactivated, too much is excreted and our oestrogen levels can fall too low. Too little oestrogen can eventually lead to diseases like obesity, metabolic syndrome, cardiovascular disease and cognitive decline. Too much oestrogen circulating around the body can lead to diseases such as endometriosis and cancer.[58]

Gut health is clearly as important for our reproductive hormones as for our long-term health. So, how do you establish a healthy gut? Before you go downing probiotic drinks like there's no tomorrow, remember the research that shows that changes to diet alone have a big impact on gut health. To encourage microbial diversity, make sure your diet contains a wide range of fruit, vegetables and fibre, and that your plate of food includes as many colours as possible – and by that we mean natural colour, such as from carrots, broccoli and sweetcorn, not cheese puffs, jelly beans and custard. Prebiotic foods such as garlic, onion, asparagus and bananas provide the material that gut bacteria like to feed on, and probiotic foods such as kefir, kombucha, kimchi and other fermented foods are really useful for introducing beneficial bacterial strains, like lactobacillus, to the gut. In case you were wondering what the difference is between probiotic and prebiotic, probiotics are foods or supplements that contain live microorganisms intended to maintain or improve the 'good' bacteria, i.e. microflora, whereas prebiotics are foods which are generally high in fibre and act as food for human microflora.

There's even evidence that being outside, getting dirty, going barefoot and touching trees can improve the variety of your gut microbiome.[59] After all, there are more microbes on a teaspoon of healthy soil than there are people on earth. But we don't need you to lick your dirty hands or eat a teaspoon of soil.[60] The healthy microbes present in soil can enter through your skin and nasal passages, so outdoor exercise in non-urban environments can have more than just the fitness benefits; it can contribute to a healthy gut, too.

To supplement or not to supplement?

Supplements are a big business – really big. But remember this: you can't supplement your way out of a bad diet. As an active woman, a poor diet – even if you decide to supplement it with the greatest vitamins and mineral tablets in the world – will impact your long- and short-term health, your feeling of vitality, and your performance in sport and exercise. A bad diet won't give you the essential carbohydrates, fats and protein needed to deliver the right amount of calories at the right time to ensure blood-sugar stability and the healthy-signalling pathway of our reproductive hormones. All of this remains compromised with a bad diet, even when accompanied by supplements. Eating well is the most effective way of reversing micronutrient deficiencies, as these are most potent when they come from food. Furthermore, food isn't just the best source of vitamins and minerals, it also gives you all the other non-essential but beneficial nutrients, such as carotenoids (which have anti-inflammatory properties), flavonoids (to protect your body against everyday toxins and stressors) and other antioxidants (which help defend your body's cells from damage), all of which aren't in most vitamin supplements. Plus, food is often much less expensive than supplements. We always recommend a 'food first' approach – try to get everything you need from the food you eat. If you feel unsure about your specific needs, then instead of spending your hard-earned money on a few months' worth of supplements, book a consultation with a dietitian to get a sense of what's missing from your diet and the changes you could consider to benefit your health and well-being.[61]

The two exceptions to the rule that nutrients should come from food, and not pills, are vitamin D and magnesium. The NHS recommends that people take a daily supplement of vitamin D during the winter to compensate for the lack of sunlight required for our body to make its own vitamin D. Magnesium, meanwhile, is vital for our overall health and well-being, yet it's often difficult to get enough through our diet, particularly as our bodies excrete magnesium as a way of dealing with stress. Since you can't test for magnesium levels, it's a case of making a judgement about your diet and lifestyle, and giving magnesium supplements a go to see if you feel better – magnesium supplementation has an effect pretty quickly. However, if you have kidney disease, magnesium supplements aren't safe for long-term use so always check with your doctor before you start taking supplements

When you opt for supplements, be aware that there can be differences between products' quality, purity, effectiveness and sustainability. In most countries, supplements are regulated as a 'food', which often has less stringent controls than medicinal or cosmetic products. Some supplements use ingredients that are more easily absorbed, faster-acting or that are filtered for greater purity. Some ingredients aren't always sourced or manufactured in a sustainable way. If you are a sportswoman who competes under anti-doping regulations, you will also need to ensure your supplements are 'batch-tested', which means tested by an independent laboratory to make sure they are free from banned substances and safe for competing athletes. Not all supplements come with this type of rigorous testing – look for an 'Informed Sport' logo to confirm independent testing has taken place.

Vegging out

There's no doubt that if you choose to adopt a vegetarian or vegan diet then it's harder to get the essential macro- and micro-nutrient supply from your food. Research shows that vegans consume less energy than omnivores and that vegetarian diets generally appear to be lower in protein, fat, vitamin B12, riboflavin, vitamin D, calcium, iron and zinc when compared with an omnivorous diet.[62] That's because animal foods really are the best source of protein, zinc, iron, and omega-3s, to name a few, and they are the only source of vitamin B12 (which helps keep the body's nerve and blood cells healthy, helps make DNA – the genetic material in all cells – and, if that wasn't enough, also helps prevent anaemia). Well-considered vegetarian diets can be sufficiently nutritious for health and performance, but the quality and timing of what you eat needs real planning. There must be an emphasis on foods fortified with iron, zinc, calcium and vitamin B12, and possibly supplementation of these key 'hot spots' for deficiencies. Vegan athletes have been shown to consume less protein than both omnivores and vegetarians. The challenge with plant-based proteins is that they are often incomplete sources of protein, missing important essential amino acids. If you're vegan, make sure you're getting good doses of protein through foods like beans, lentils, tofu, nuts, seeds and most grains, including quinoa; and if you're vegetarian, choose milk, Greek yoghurt, cottage cheese and eggs for your protein. When you suspect that you aren't getting enough calories from a vegan or vegetarian diet, a good strategy is to increase how often you eat and to up your intake of energy-dense foods such as nuts, seeds and oils.

We pass no judgement on being vegan or vegetarian, but we do urge you to acknowledge that this dietary approach can come at a cost, particularly for very active women. Getting regular, quality protein to support training and adaptation, making sure your micronutrient intake supports hormone health and that your overall energy intake is sufficient and not sending you into energy deficit, is more challenging if you are vegan or vegetarian. Despite the hype, there is no evidence that there are performance gains to be had from this approach to eating, and because of the likelihood of undereating on these types of diets, the risk of energy deficiency and its impact on performance may be increased. By being conscientious and organized, you can happily eat lots of nutrient-dense plant-based meals with enough protein, fat and minerals such as zinc and calcium. But being conscientious and organized isn't for everyone, and certainly not for teenagers, who in our experience base their vegetarian diet around cheese and pasta. So if you have adopted or are thinking of adopting this approach, or your teenage daughters/nieces/friends are doing so, then please be diligent in making sure that you fully support your, or their, sport and activities through a well-balanced diet.

The magic formula for diets

Is there such a thing as the 'best' diet – the way we should all be eating to stay healthy, happy, fit and high-performing throughout life? No. You know the three of us well enough by now to know that we fully believe this, because every woman is different, and every woman's body in the context of her sport, her relationships, her work, her life, is different. Added to the fact that your nutritional needs change when you go through periods of more or less exercise training, or when your training goals change, we couldn't possibly design a generic meal plan that would work for you all. But we also believe that getting nutrition right shouldn't be complicated. Here are our guiding principles for active women:

- Take in enough energy to fuel your training and busy lifestyle. That means getting enough calories and delivering them to your hard-working body at regular intervals throughout the day so it never thinks it's going to starve.
- Make sure you have a good balance of macronutrients – about 55% carbs, 20% fat and 25% protein over the course of your day.
- Meet the needs of your training as it changes – for example, more strength work means your protein load should go up a bit to help with recovery and adaptation of muscle.
- Limit processed foods to treats, not staples, and eat a variety of foods including lots of veg – which should ensure you are getting an adequate supply of important micronutrients and are creating a lovely diverse microbiome in your gut.

As long as you take this approach, the detail is up to you. What's really important is that you enjoy your food – don't be afraid of it; don't be worried about having an appetite – as an active woman, that is your body asking for fuel. The food you eat really is the fuel you need to be the best version of yourself, whether that's running around after the kids, or chasing down that PB. Food is fuel and can help training and performance. It can also be medicine, helping you feel better and happier, and to live longer. Put good stuff in, and you'll get good stuff out (and we're not just talking better poos – but yes, that too).

Waving a RED-S flag

Relative energy deficiency in sport (RED-S) is something every active woman should be aware of, because it's a clear red flag that something is going wrong with your health and well-being, and that you need to do something about it. Energy deficiency can be caused by undereating, over-training (or a combination of both), or for reasons like emotional stress or trauma. Signs of RED-S include:

- weight loss or being underweight
- periods stopping or becoming irregular
- recurrent illnesses, e.g. colds and flus
- decreased sports performance
- mood changes
- delayed/disordered growth or development (in children and teenagers)
- iron deficiency
- mental health conditions (e.g. depression or anxiety)[63]

Since 2014, when researchers in this field of work published the first consensus statement on RED-S, explaining its causes and its effects on athletes, progress has been made in understanding the consequences for active women who go for long periods of time not fuelling well enough to meet the energy demands of their active life.[64] These consequences are now known to apply to the whole body and affect physical, psychological and emotional health, as well as impacting a woman's ability to train, adapt and perform in sport and exercise. In addition to having physical symptoms, it's very common for women who are under-fuelling to suffer from mental health challenges, and there is a much greater risk of depression in those suffering from RED-S.

Emma

A few years ago, I mentored some aspiring sports scientists who were researching female athlete health for their PhDs. In one of our first meetings, I asked the women to share their story of what had led them to be interested in pursuing research on women's health in sport. One of the women, Jen, floored me with her story. In her early teens she had developed the eating disorder anorexia. She hid the extent of her condition, and started to have a very successful running career, moving through the ranks towards national representation. But by the time she was twenty she couldn't hide her condition any more and became so ill that she was treated in an inpatient unit for several months. After years of malnutrition, her bones were riddled with osteoporosis – the bone-weakening condition that usually affects women in their eighties, not a twenty-one-year-old. She had used her relationship with food as a means of coping and controlling her life. While treatment gradually restored her bodyweight, the recovery of her mental health is still ongoing. But her experiences motivated her to pursue a PhD in RED-S and to improve awareness of the condition so that coaches and athletes alike understand the signs and symptoms, and the significance of ignoring them.

I've taught athletes and coaches about RED-S for many years and worked with athletes who lost their periods because they weren't fuelling their training effectively, but this was generally unintentional under-fuelling, which we were able to redress through attention to diet and the timing of meals. Jen was the first person I met who had, due to her eating disorder, ignored her body's warnings, including the loss of her periods, and continued to undereat and over-train, and was now living with the devastating consequences, not just for her participation in sport, but her lifelong health. Jen's wasn't the only story I would hear from athletes who had been broken by an ambitious pursuit of sporting goals coupled with the sporting culture that believes a light, lean body, at all costs, is the only way to be competitive.

The reason periods stop when someone is suffering from RED-S is because, when the body lacks energy, one of the first things it can do to save energy, without compromising its ability to survive, is to switch off our reproductive system. We need our cardiovascular system, our nervous system and our immune system to live. But our reproductive system is not essential to taking our next breath, or even staying upright over the next few days or weeks. Periods stopping happens alongside many other malfunctions in the body, which are less easy to spot because they aren't marked by something as obvious as having, or not having, a period bleed. Not all women who have RED-S will lose their periods completely: instead, cycles may become irregular, and periods heavier with worse symptoms. If the menstrual cycle is a window into our overall health and well-being, the menstrual cycle of someone suffering from RED-S will reflect that. RED-S is not just menstrual cycle dysfunction and the catastrophic

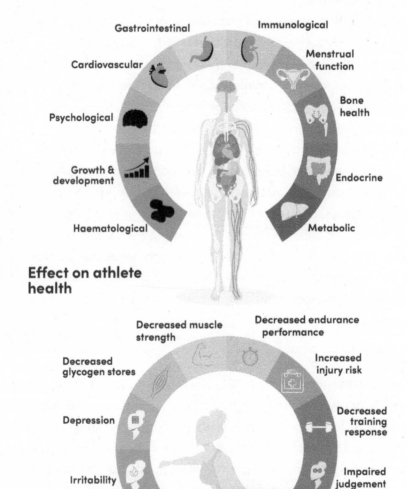

Effect on athlete health

Effect on athlete performance

The consequence of RED-S for our health and for our exercise and sports performance consequence of hormonal loss that women experience, it also impacts women at a psychological level, and affects their immune function, digestive function, metabolic function . . . the list goes on.

As you might imagine, RED-S is more prevalent in weight-managed sports, where bodyweight is an important determinant of success, and coaches and athletes believe that 'lighter is faster' – which it is, until it's not. Athletes need to be light and healthy to be successful, and often, those two things don't go hand-in-hand. RED-S affects a larger proportion of women in sports where what we look like is an important element of per-formance, such as gymnastics and dance, or for girls who feel societal or social media pressure to be a certain shape or size. For example, in one study, 100% of the college cheerleaders in the study had RED-S.[65] But it's important to note that RED-S can happen in any active woman; they don't have to look very thin, nor appear to be restricting their eating. A lot of the time RED-S is unintentional – it may happen when an increase in training load isn't matched with an appropriately timed increase of nutritional intake. Or it can be that the athlete is underestimat-ing other sources of energy expenditure outside of training, like cycling to work or school, or even the energy demands of school or work itself. Look out for when increases in your training load are accompanied by weight loss, inability to recover, constant fatigue, or a lack of progression in fitness or strength that you would usually expect given the training you're doing.

Sometimes RED-S can occur because of the intentional restriction of energy intake through dieting, and this can be linked to an eating disorder. Eating disorders are complex condi-tions and are caused by a combination of social, physical and emotional factors. A discussion of these is outside the scope of this book, but if you think you may have an unhealthy relation-ship with food and your body image, firstly know you are not alone, and secondly know that help is available – please reach out for it. Clinical dietitians are trained to support eating disorders.

Baz

Before I rowed, I was a high-jumper. My coach insisted that I should weigh less than 60kg (which may sound reasonable, but I'm 6ft, so no, it's not). I started training more and eating less – it was a vicious circle, but I genuinely didn't know what else to do or how to stop, despite the fact that my performance started to plummet. My periods had stopped but I didn't say anything. Everyone around me seemed to be managing this much training, so I just figured I'd do the same. I eventually went to see a doctor – but I wasn't thin enough to be considered anorexic, and since I never mentioned my relationship with food I was put on the pill and sent away. I stopped high-jumping because it all became too miserable. I very slowly got myself back on track with my food, but it took years. I am very grateful to have found rowing, which, despite its arduous training programmes, is a sport where strong, powerful females are looked up to, and I found myself training with women who were not restricting their intake at all, or obsessing about food, and I wanted to be like them!

We must be brave in holding coaches, teachers or trainers to account for the language they use. Whether it's giving a correction about skill that could be misinterpreted as an insult to body shape, or imparting judgement on body size, we need to call this out when we see it, to stop the risk of active women restricting their nutrition and suffering both physically and emotionally as a consequence.

RED-S is far too prevalent among active girls and women. We need to inform coaches and teachers about it, we need to educate girls about the power of food or lack of it, and to raise awareness of the signs and symptoms to look out for. We need to reframe societal attitudes towards food and body shape.

The fact that RED-S is such a common problem demonstrates the structural inadequacies across sport and physical activity. Here's what we think needs to happen to change that.

Stop:

- normalizing the loss of periods in active women as something that 'just happens if you train hard enough'
- directing athletes to the pill to 'kick-start' their menstrual cycle
- weighing and measuring active women and girls too often – with too much emphasis placed on size and shape over form and function
- food being restricted or judgement placed upon what and how much active women eat
- silence when there's obviously a problem. We can't just turn a blind eye to very underweight women, signs of disordered eating or recurrent injury and illness. We need to be prepared to lean into difficult conversations, with compassion

Start:

- implementing and supporting qualifications to include information on RED-S as standard for all teachers, coaches, physios and personal trainers – indeed, all those involved in the sports industry
- education for athletes, active women and parents on female-focused nutrition
- well-defined referral pathways to accessible specialists including clinical dietitians, qualified sports nutritionists, psychologists and psychotherapists

- regular female-focused health screening as part of any sports programme or sporting system to recognize those women who might not be getting their nutrition right, or have menstrual cycle dysfunction as a consequence of RED-S
- doctors being taught about RED-S as an essential part of professional development training

How do I know if I am in energy deficit?

If you want to really check in on whether you're getting sufficient energy from your food to meet the demands of your training and your life, you can work out what's called your 'energy availability' – or EA, measured in kcal per kg of your fat-free mass – FFM – per day.[66] This calculation takes into account the energy you get from your diet, the energy you expend while exercising and the energy you have left to perform all the bodily functions required to live your life. The concept was first studied in women, and the researchers established that if they had an EA of forty-five, they were likely taking in enough energy for optimal health, but if their EA fell below thirty for too long, women experienced impairments of a variety of body functions, which we now associate with RED-S.

To calculate your EA

1. Calculate your daily energy intake in kcal, based on the food you eat. You'll likely have to use an app to record what you eat, and this will calculate your total calories consumed in a day.
2. Calculate your FFM by multiplying your bodyweight, in kg, by your body-fat percentage, which is measured using a skinfold test or bioelectrical scales. You should be able to get your body fat measured at the doctors, your gym or by using home scales with this feature.
3. Calculate the energy you expend during your training or

exercise in kcal (you'll need the help of a smart watch, heart-rate monitor or fitness tracker for this).

4. Subtract the energy you expend in kcal during your training from your energy intake in kcal.

5. Divide this number by your FFM to get your EA.

Example EA calculation

A woman's bodyweight is 60kg and she has 20% body fat.

She therefore has 12kg of body fat ($60 \times 0.20 = 12$), so her FFM is $60 - 12 = 48$kg.

Her energy intake is 2800kcal per day.

Her exercise energy demands are 800kcal per day.

Her energy availability, or EA, is therefore ($2800 - 800 = 2000$) $\div 48 = 41$ kcal/kg FFM per day.

How to eat well

- Unleash the power of food by eating a well-balanced diet to suit your active lifestyle.
- Eat regularly throughout the day to give your body the energy to perform and adapt to training, and your hormones what they need to be healthy – no fasted training or long periods without food.
- Don't consider supplementing until you've had a good, honest look at whether your diet could be better.
- Remember that good eating behaviour is reliant on having access to the right food at the right time.
- Understand the signs, symptoms and consequences of undereating and/or over-training.
- Be part of a culture that sees food as fuel and not something to limit or restrict. Be a role model for those around you, and generations to follow, to look up to.

Chapter 9

Sleeping Well

We all love our sleep. Most of us have learned that when we regularly experience a lack of sleep, it can really impact our daily lives. While the research into the importance of sleep for active people and athletes has increased significantly over the past decade, and there are various articles on why women need more sleep than men, there's little specifically considering sleep in active women.[1] We realize that some of you may work shifts, and as a result sleep during the day and work at night, but for simplicity's sake, what follows is based mainly on the routine of wakeful days and sleepy nights.

At The Well HQ, our experience has shown us that sleep is a topic that cannot be ignored, even if the gender-specific data isn't always available. Exercise can actually put you at risk of getting less sleep, depending on the time of day you exercise and your workout intensity.[2] Doing a Yin yoga class at 8 p.m. at night has a very different effect on your sleep when compared with a late-night workout at CrossFit. But while being active might sometimes compromise your sleep, there's plenty of evidence that the amount and quality of your sleep can support and even improve your health, fitness and performance.[3] Focusing on sleep is a total no-brainer – if you nail it, it's a free performance boost. As an elite athlete, Baz was always looking for gains which didn't require her to put more effort into actual training. The non-training components of your life – including sleep, nutrition and psychology – are great ways to give yourself an edge.

Why is sleep so important for active women?

On every level, sleep is a total winner. Rest and recovery are vital components of any well-designed training programme. Let's take repair and growth of muscle, which is an essential part of our recovery and adaptation process as we train and get fitter. The release of growth hormone, which is a key element of this repair and growth process, is greatly enhanced during sleep. While the impact of not sleeping well can accrue over time, even a single night of restricted sleep after a heavy exercise session was found to result in a 4% decrease in performance the following morning among cyclists.[4] In short, you simply won't recover or adapt as well if you don't get good sleep.[5]

When it comes to actual sports performance, the bulk of available research focuses on men, and we have to hypothesize which of these studies could likely also apply to women.[6] When male basketball players increased their sleep by two hours per night for about six weeks, a study found significant improvements in sprint times, as well as players reporting feeling less fatigued during practices and games.[7] For endurance exercise, lack of sleep can make the same workout feel harder.[8] Researchers found that in a thirty-minute treadmill test, male participants were able to run less far after a night of sleep deprivation, compared with a night of normal sleep. Their physiological responses during running were the same during each trial, which led the researchers to suggest that a more psychological effect may have been slowing them down.[9]

In skill-based sports, lack of sleep seems to have some of the most significant effects on reaction time and accuracy. In tennis, for example, after a night of sleep deprivation (defined as a night with five hours of sleep), players' serving accuracy worsened by 53% compared with an individual's normal night's sleep (which on average was seven and three quarter hours).[10] This study included women, and the female players' accuracy was more affected by lack of sleep than the male players'. In other tennis research, when players had about ninety minutes' sleep extra per night for a week, their serving accuracy improved by 41%.[11] It's not more practice you need, it's more sleep!

Getting enough sleep also reduces the risk of injury in athletes. Research shows that those who get fewer than eight hours per night are 70% more likely to report an injury than those who get more sleep than this.[12] Interestingly, the greatest risk of injury is when training load increases and sleep decreases. How many of us are guilty of sacrificing sleep during busy times, just to cram in extra training alongside work and home life? Sacrificing sleep isn't a long-term solution for fitting everything in.[13]

How much sleep do athletes need?

The basic principles of sleep are the same for everyone: we all sleep in cycles of roughly ninety minutes, with adults requiring between seven and nine hours of sleep for optimal performance and health, and adolescents requiring more, ideally between eight and ten hours. In his best-selling book, *Why We Sleep*, Matthew Walker sets out a very strong case for adults getting at least eight hours of sleep per night,[14] while other research, this time from Cambridge University, suggests that seven hours is an optimal amount for those in middle age.[15] Whatever number you go with, everyone, especially active women, should be aiming for seven to eight hours a night to realize the health and exercise benefits.[16]

From a neurophysiological point of view, an active woman's sleep is the same as anyone else's, but the challenges to getting good sleep can be different. Some sports, like rowing or swimming, may require you to be up early to train, or you might only have time to work out before your day gets going. You may enjoy an evening exercise class or have club training scheduled after work to suit most members. Each of these factors – having to get up early or doing a late training session – poses a threat to getting a good night's sleep.[17] Even an increase in training load can negatively impact sleep. Research found that when the amount of exercise you're doing increases by more than 25%, it results in a decrease in total sleep time. This is thought to be due to increased levels of stress hormones brought about by the extra training. This is ironic, because the more exercise you're doing, the more your body will need sleep for the processes of recovery and adaptation.[18] But when stress hormones are high, it can impact both the onset of sleep and its quality. As we at The Well HQ always say, knowledge is empowering. Knowing that when your training schedule ramps up, or when you're training late in the evening or early in the morning, you're more likely to suffer the negative impact of lack of sleep, then you can make an effort to address that. You might adjust your bedtime, make an extra effort to follow a bedtime routine, or set your alarm a bit later.

Sleepiness saps motivation

While it makes perfect sense, we sometimes forget how feeling tired can really impact our get-up-and-go, and there's good evidence that having too little sleep can influence your motivation to exercise. In a study of more than 10,000 older women, those who reported getting fewer than seven hours of sleep a night spent the most time being sedentary the following day and performed relatively little moderate-to-vigorous exercise.[19] Meanwhile, those who had the highest levels of physical activity (at least twenty minutes of moderate-to-vigorous movement) on a given day were most likely to have had seven to nine hours' sleep that night. If you wonder where your motivation to train or your enthusiasm to exercise has gone, it's worth checking your sleeping habits.

Cat naps

Where schedules allow, napping can be an effective way to bank more sleep, keep fatigue at bay and regain your motivation to move again. There's a knack to napping, though, and getting the timing and duration of a nap right can ensure it has restorative powers, rather than leaving you feeling worse than you started.

Nap time

- The optimal time of day for napping, which really suits the body's daily biological rhythm, is between midday and 4 p.m.[20] During this time, we have a temporary dip in our core temperature, which is a great cue for sleepiness.
- It's best to stick to either twenty or ninety minutes for a nap.[21] A nap duration of up to twenty minutes is considered optimal to avoid slow-wave or deep sleep. Alternatively, ninety minutes is also considered optimal as this allows a complete sleep cycle including both NREM, or non-REM, and REM sleep to occur. The sleep cycle includes four stages, the first three of which are NREM, the fourth REM sleep. The third NREM stage is the deep sleep stage that kicks in after about twenty minutes of sleep and is the period when your body repairs and regrows tissues, builds bone and muscle, and strengthens the immune system. REM sleep is generally when you dream. Waking up during the third stage of deeper sleep can lead to you feeling worse when you wake up. The technical term for this grogginess is sleep inertia.

- Don't nap too close to bedtime. During the day, we build up a need to sleep, and that's what drives good sleep at night. If we have a nap late in the afternoon, it's like having a snack just before dinner – it takes the edge off that sleep need and reduces our sleepiness, which can mean we go to bed later or have trouble falling asleep.[22]
- Naps don't suit everyone, nor are they necessary – if your night-time sleep is sufficient, that's great. But if you're not getting enough sleep at night, then short naps can be an excellent way to top up your daily sleep deficit.
- Naps can improve performance. In a study of match-day naps in New Zealand netballers, scores on a jump test and the coach's rating of match performance were better in the players who'd had a twenty-minute nap earlier in the day.[23]

Quality is as important as quantity

Noticing the quality of your sleep is just as important as ensuring you get enough of it. Sleep quality is reflected in how satisfied you are with your sleep: can you fall asleep easily, can you sleep for a solid eight hours, or, if roused, can you get back to sleep easily and do you feel refreshed when you wake up? We're all aware of things that affect our quality of our sleep, even if they don't impact on how long we sleep. It's easy to fall asleep and get eight hours in bed after a few glasses of wine, but the quality of that sleep is certainly impaired. We might feel tired after an intense workout and go to bed early, but restless legs and twitchy, aching muscles impact how well we sleep during the night. Stress can also stop us from drifting off to sleep or keep us awake during the night.

As with all things related to simple statements like 'get more, and better, sleep', there may be some digging to do to find what's really impacting your ability to do that. Going to bed at a reasonable time in the evening to ensure you can get a full seven or eight hours sleep before your alarm clock goes off the next morning helps, but the things that affect the quality of your sleep might be more subtle, or totally unrelated to your night-time activities. What you do in the day – what you eat, what's going on at work, your training, stress and your ability to manage it – can all show up at night, when you're trying to get your well-earned rest.

One less sleep

Perhaps you're so nervous the night before a game that you toss and turn, and can't get a good night's sleep. Perhaps a deadline at work is playing on your mind, stopping you from falling asleep quickly. Or perhaps the children invaded your bed at 2 a.m. because of a bad dream. There are many times when, no matter how much we want to get a good night's sleep before a big day, we can't. The good news is that, for the most part, your performance is unlikely to be detrimentally affected because of this. There are exceptions: if you're in the middle of a tournament and need to recover from one big game in order to compete in another tomorrow, then impaired sleep can mean impaired recovery. Or if you participate in a highly skilled sport that relies on precise accuracy, like archery or tennis, then lack of sleep can affect the finesse of your performance. Other than that, we're capable of performing to our potential across a range of activities with the odd night of poor sleep.[24] If you're struggling to sleep, the best thing to do is not worry about it. It's easier said than done, as you toss and turn, knowing how important sleep is. If you know that you're likely to suffer from poor sleep the night before the big day because you have a tendency to get nervous, then just accept it and do everything you can to sleep well during the week leading up to the night before – before your nerves get the better of you.

So many sleepless nights

One night's poor sleep may not hurt, but an extended period of insufficient or poor-quality sleep can have a detrimental effect on short- and long-term health. It's called chronic sleep loss and it can impair memory by 20%, reaction time by 25% and communication by 30%, and it can cause athletes to be less able to deal with new situations or learn new things.[25] A study of people who had sleep apnoea, which had affected their quality of sleep over a long period of time, showed they were five times more likely than people getting enough sleep to be involved in a car accident. Researchers used insurance records to look at the nature of the car accidents, and of the small number of truly awful crashes – head-on collisions and collisions with pedestrians or cyclists – 80% involved the sleep apnoea patients.[26] Driving while sleep-deprived can have the same effects as driving while over the alcohol limit, which gives you an idea of what sleep loss does to our brains.[27]

The health consequences of poor sleep for prolonged periods of time go beyond a greater chance of being in a car accident, though. Simply put, lack of sleep leads to a shorter life.[28] Poor sleepers have an increased risk of diabetes, cardiovascular disease and mental illness, and research suggests that women are more susceptible to the effects of chronic sleep loss than men are. Women have also been found to be more susceptible to high blood pressure, weight gain and depression as a consequence of sleep deprivation.[29]

Women's sleep

There's an interesting dichotomy in women's sleep: women need more sleep than men, but they are more likely to suffer from insomnia. Women need on average twenty minutes more sleep per day than men, and research suggests – as clichéd as this sounds – that this is because women are more likely to multitask and use more of their brain throughout the day.[30] The more you use your brain during the day, the more sleep it will need.

Despite this need for more sleep, women are actually 40% more likely to suffer insomnia than men and are more likely to have sleep problems.[31] There are a number of reasons for this poorer sleep in women, one being that we are more likely to ruminate and worry, which stops us from falling asleep.[32] We don't have to be at the mercy of our biological sex here. There are strategies we can employ that are shown to reduce rumination and anxiety, so if that's stopping you from falling asleep each night, take action! One of the best things you can do is switch off your phone an hour before bedtime, which not only ensures that our brain biology is not disrupted by the blue light emitted by the phone's screen (which basically tricks us into thinking it's still daytime), but also helps you avoid mindless social media or news scrolling, WhatsApp groups from school or work, and email, which can all trigger rumination.[33]

Another reason women may be more likely to suffer from insomnia is that we are twice as likely to suffer with restless legs syndrome, which causes unpleasant or uncomfortable sensations in the legs and an irresistible urge to move them.[34] Symptoms commonly occur in the late afternoon or evening, and are often most severe at night, when you're resting, either sitting or lying in bed, which is why it interferes so much with sleep. Restless legs syndrome can be genetic and is understood to be linked to how the body handles dopamine, which controls muscle movement,[35] but it has also been linked to iron deficiency. As we've mentioned, women have a greater risk of iron deficiency and anaemia, and this can manifest itself in restless legs. If you're suffering from this, go and see your doctor, as there are things you can do to alleviate the symptoms. Get your iron checked for a start, but also start working out what triggers the restlessness;

alcohol, muscle soreness or medications such as antihistamines and antidepressants can all cause restless legs. If necessary, you can try medications that might help, on the advice of your doctor.

The menstrual sleep cycle

We established that women's hormones fluctuate across the menstrual cycle. This fluctuation can help or hinder your sleep, depending on where in your cycle you are. Once progesterone starts to rise, in the second half of the cycle, after ovulation, it improves your sleep by helping you fall asleep more quickly and supporting better-quality, restorative sleep.[36] If you're tracking your cycle, you might be able to make a concerted effort to get to bed at a decent time in that third week, knowing your body is on your side and supporting good sleep. Although progesterone aids sleep, it also increases your body temperature by up to half a degree. Since a slight dip in body temperature is generally our cue for sleep at bedtime, any rise in core temperature, such as the one caused by progesterone in the second half of our cycle, can blunt the effectiveness of this signal. Most of the time, once we've fallen asleep, a further decrease in core temperature promotes deeper sleep, but if you're running hotter because you're in the luteal phase or are suffering from hot flushes due to the menopause, you might find this knocks your sleep off track too. Try to keep your bedroom cooler, which can help your body to cool down enough to reach a level of deeper, restorative sleep. Interestingly, research has shown that night-time body temperature is higher in women taking the pill, because the synthetic progestins have a similar effect on body temperature as progesterone in a natural cycle.[37]

When oestrogen and progesterone start to fall, at the end of your cycle, in the premenstrual phase, sleep becomes lighter and may be more disturbed. PMS symptoms such as pain and anxiety may also interfere with sleep, making poor sleep another symptom of PMS. Women with PMS have self-reported experiencing an increase in unpleasant dreams, night-time awakenings and morning tiredness in comparison with women without PMS.[38] It's a vicious circle, really, as lack of sleep at this time can also intensify premenstrual symptoms and premenstrual dysphoric disorder (PMDD). So, you can't sleep because of PMS, but your lack of sleep is making your PMS worse. Wonderful!

Simply knowing about your sleep across your cycle is an important step. When you track cycle symptoms, make sure you include particularly good or bad sleep in your tracking, too, as it might help you identify when you need to be paying more attention to your pre-bedtime routine and sleep habits, and when you can take advantage of when your body finds good sleep easier to come by.

Pausing sleep during the menopause

Sleep disturbances are common in older women, affecting 40–60% of perimenopausal or postmenopausal women. Indeed, sleep issues are considered a core symptom of menopause.[39] During this phase of life, women wake more frequently in the night and tend to have poorer sleep quality, which can have an effect on daytime alertness, clarity of thought and mental health. It's unknown whether other symptoms of the menopause cause sleep issues, such as hot flushes and anxiety, or whether the hormonal changes happening at menopause are themselves responsible for the challenges to sleep. As with all things hormonal, it's likely a complex combination of all these factors. Hormone replacement therapy has been shown to improve sleep quality by reducing symptoms such as hot flushes and night sweats, as well as by regulating hormone levels.[40]

Don't give up on sleep

Women who are pregnant, have recently given birth or have small children, or who are perimenopausal or postmenopausal, will, without a doubt, find their sleep is impacted at these times of life. If you're one of those women that has just written yourself off as a poor sleeper or given up on the chances of ever sleeping well again – don't do that! Sleep is too fundamental and important to give up on – there is always hope and something that can be done. But when you're exhausted and sleep-deprived, it really is difficult to see how you might be able to resolve the situation. It may not be possible to rectify it straight away, but developing strategies that might help, and prioritizing getting your sleep back on track, is essential for your short- and long-term health and happiness. You need to have some good sleep back in your life.

Clean up your sleep hygiene

Good sleep hygiene – the things you do in the lead-up to bedtime – can often be enough to rectify sleep problems, with 30% of people overcoming their sleep issues just by making improvements to their sleep hygiene.[41] Here are our top tips for getting a good night's sleep.

- Keep a cool bedroom (18 degrees Celsius is optimal).
- Keep your bedroom dark. If you can't, channel your inner Audrey Hepburn and wear an eye mask.
- Ban screens before bed, or by the bed (buy an old-school alarm clock) and leave your devices charging in another room.
- Have a bedtime routine, including things that relax and soothe you. (If you have young kids, think of what you do with them: bath, story, lullaby – this routine is there to settle them and signal that it's time for bed. Adults need this as well.)

- Make sure you're exposed to light in the day, ideally sunlight. Light and dark are the biggest drivers of our circadian rhythm, our sleep–wake cycle.
- Manage your caffeine intake – ideally none after midday.
- Limit your alcohol intake – it might make it easier to fall asleep in the first place, but it makes staying asleep much harder.
- Don't eat too late as this means your digestive system will still be working hard when your body is trying to get to sleep.
- Don't exercise too late, to prevent those endorphins that put you on a natural high after training and stop your body from winding down. Ideally, you should aim to end your training two to three hours before bed so that your body has time to wind down and switch off before you try to sleep. If you have to exercise at night, try a longer cool-down to help you decompress.
- Have a warm bath or shower before bed to help you relax.
- Try some breathing exercises or meditation to help you access your parasympathetic (calming) nervous system.
- Try and wake up at the same time each morning – it helps to improve sleep quality by reinforcing a consistent sleep–wake cycle. If you get this right, you'll be able to ditch the alarm clock completely and your body will wake naturally.[42]
- If you're eating late at night after getting back from your workout, make sure you have quick access to easily digestible food such as yoghurt and berries, porridge with peanut butter and banana, or nuts and seeds – all of which are snacks that have been shown to promote better sleep.[43]

Sleeping pills

Imagine you've not slept properly for weeks. You know how beneficial sleep is and yet, when you go to bed, you just can't switch off your mind. You lie there until 3 a.m. thinking about all the reasons why you should be sleeping. Finally, at 4 a.m., you fall asleep – and within two hours it's time to wake up and get on with your day. You feel physically terrible and you're already worrying about whether you'll be able to sleep that night. Those suffering from this type of sleepless scenario often ask their doctor for sleeping pills to help them get to sleep. This is particularly the case for athletes, whose use of sleep medication is higher than in the general population. When Baz was rowing for Britain, many of her teammates took sleeping pills, which helped them in the short term but failed to get to the root cause of the issue to achieve a long-term solution, which is not a healthy approach.[44]

Sleeping pills do have a place in the world of medicine and there are times when a doctor will prescribe them. But drugs should be used as a last resort, and of course the female filter needs to be applied, as women metabolize these drugs differently than men do and tend to have significantly higher levels of the medication in their blood even eight hours after taking it. Sleeping pills can also be addictive. An unusual silver-medal performance by Australian swimmer Grant Hackett at the 2008 Olympics (he had won two golds in the previous Games and was expected to do the same in 2008) led people to suggest the sleeping pill he was taking was to blame. Hackett described taking sleeping pills to a point of 'heavy reliance' during his recovery from a shoulder surgery and to help with rest during competition.[45] Due to the addictive nature and possible side effects, the Australian Olympic Committee now bans the use of sleeping pills for its athletes as soon as they have been selected for an Olympic team.[46]

It's important to look at the underlying causes of your insomnia and to explore non-medication options such as lifestyle changes, through your sleep hygiene, and stress management. Taking sleeping pills can be a short-term solution, but taken for the long-term, they can create more problems of their own and leave the root cause of your insomnia unknown.

In addition to adopting good sleep hygiene, one treatment that can help if you continue to suffer from sleeplessness is cognitive behavioural therapy for insomnia (CBT-I), which in the UK is available on the NHS.[47] In fact, CBT-I has been found to be the most effective treatment for chronic insomnia and is better than medication in terms of effectiveness and long-term benefits.[48] It uses various different methods, including improvements to sleep hygiene, plus sleep restriction, relaxation training and other mindfulness-based approaches.

Go to sleep!

There's no shortage of advice on how to improve your sleep, but one thing is for sure: each one of us finds some strategies more helpful than others, or that fit better into our daily routine. Find what works for you, but do make getting enough, good-quality sleep one of your health and well-being priorities. The following are our top tips for getting it right.

Listen to your body

Dr Luke Gupta is a sports physiologist who specializes in sleep and works with Olympic and Paralympic athletes. He suggests that one of the best things a person can do to get a good night's sleep is to go to bed when you feel sleepy.[49] Sounds simple, doesn't it? But we often stick to a very strict bedtime or we count back eight hours from the time we need to wake up and set our bedtime accordingly. Going to bed before you're sleepy is like sitting down to dinner before you're hungry, your body just isn't ready yet. Then, when you fail to fall asleep, you become anxious about not getting enough sleep, and can end up in a sleeplessness spiral.

Feeling sleepy at the end of the day is our body's way of saying it's ready to sleep, and it's a great cue that you should be heading off to bed.

Data is queen

Sleep diaries can help you understand whether you're getting enough sleep and, if not, what's impacting your sleep.[50] They can highlight erratic sleep patterns, your personal triggers for a bad night's sleep, and the things that help you sleep well. Dr Bella had a visit from a woman struggling to sleep, and it was only after completing a sleep diary for a week that the reason became clear: she was drinking a cappuccino after work to perk her up before her evening Pilates class. Caffeine can stay in your system for four to six hours, so having a cup of coffee in the afternoon or evening means it will still be in your system when you go to bed. We recommend avoiding caffeine or having decaffeinated coffee from midday onwards.

Use your sleep diary to record how much sleep you get each night and give yourself a score out of ten for the soundness and quality of your sleep. Ask yourself the following:

- How many times are you getting up in the night to go to the toilet? Once is fine, but are you able to get back to sleep quickly after you've been?
- Are you so concerned about your hydration that you're downing a pint of water before bed and then finding that you're up all night, back and forth to the toilet?
- Is your pelvic floor strength impacting your sleep? A weak pelvic floor can affect bladder control. Doing regular pelvic floor exercises may help improve your sleep.
- Is your menstrual cycle impacting your sleep pattern (which it can do simply by making you hotter during the second half of your cycle)?

- If you take a step back and look at your life – your work life, your home life, your training – are you asking too much of yourself?
- Are you stressed about work, money or relationships?
- Are there upcoming events on your mind?
- Do you have any feelings of anxiety or depression?

Try to understand your sleeping pattern as much as possible in order to identify what may be impacting your ability to sleep well. But make sure that the way you monitor and record your sleep doesn't stress you out even more. Recent reports have shown that, for some, monitoring sleep actually causes them to have less sleep![51]

What do you do when you have the answers to these questions?

Once you've drilled down and have a good understanding of your sleeping patterns and what may be stopping you getting enough quality sleep, you can start to address those issues. Sleep is a very personal, multifaceted and complex thing, and a generalized approach is unlikely to suit you. When you're an active woman, it's not simply about following a series of sleep hygiene rules – it goes much further than that. It's about being able to acknowledge that you're tired and that the current set-up is not working for you, and not being judged for that but instead trying to work out sustainable strategies to overcome your sleeplessness. Making sure you're sleeping well as an active woman means being holistic and being able to talk openly about all the things that could be affecting your sleep, so that you can address those issues and get on with being your best self and doing what you need to do to achieve your goals.

How to sleep well

- There's no badge of honour for existing on very little sleep – sleep is when the body does some of its best work. Make sure sleep makes it to the top of your to-do list.
- Actively create environments where you can get good sleep and develop habits that you keep as a matter of course in the lead-up to bedtime.
- If you're chronically exhausted, something needs to change. Either you're doing too much or not sleeping enough. Be honest with yourself.
- Get to the bottom of your poor sleep by using a sleep diary. Rumination, hot flushes or bladder issues, for example, will each require very different approaches to improve things.
- Exercise is great for making us sleep better, but if you're exercising early in the morning or late at night, check whether it's impacting your sleep. If it is, don't stop exercising, but develop ways to limit its negative impact on your quality or quantity of sleep.

Chapter 10

A Woman's Brain

The myth of the gendered brain

There are so many clichés around the male and female brain: women are more emotional, great at multitasking, and less likely to go for promotions or ask for pay rises, versus men, who are good at DIY jobs, map reading, computer coding, and aggressively climbing corporate ladders. We haven't met anyone who doesn't have an opinion on what the differences are in the way women and men think and behave. This 'difference' is exacerbated in the sport and exercise setting because sport is still a male-dominated system, designed originally by men, for men, and the coach–athlete or personal trainer–client relationship is often male–female.

Men are becoming increasingly open about the fact that they find it difficult to know how best to engage with the active women they coach or train, and this factor is recognized as a key barrier to participation, engagement and progression in girls and women in sport.[1] As the well-known book title suggests, sometimes it really does feel like men are from Mars and women are from Venus. But far from being totally alien to one another in the way we think, the emerging consensus by neuroscientists is that there is no such thing as a male and a female brain.[2] Forensic scientists can use teeth and bones to determine someone's sex, but if they scooped a brain out of someone's head and inspected it, they wouldn't be able to tell the difference.

Our amazing brain is sculpted by genes, hormones and biology – that's the nature bit. It's also affected by childhood experiences, education, social connections, culture and the world around us – the nurture bit. Which means that no two brains end up the same, because we all have a unique combination of nature and nurture. In fact, no brain 'ends up' like anything at all. Our brains are 'plastic', which means they are continually responding to every experience we have, and the trillions of connections that make up our brain are constantly rewiring, shaped by our environment and experiences, until we die.[3]

However, rather than everyone simply being beautifully unique, research also shows that, on average, brains have some characteristics relating to thought and behaviour that are more commonly seen in females than males. Some of this is down to different neurophysiology – the way blood flows and electrical signals transmit through our brains – and some (probably a lot) of this is down to how males and females are influenced differently by culture, our experiences and societal norms. So, there's no such thing as a female or male brain. Except that there is. Kind of. Brilliant. That's settled then.

The challenge is that brains are hugely complex, and there's still lots we don't understand about them. And the human experience is equally complex, and there's still lots we don't understand about that, either. So, to clumsily classify everyone with a female brain as being like 'this' and everyone with a male brain as being like 'that' is both unrealistic and unhelpful. But we can avoid oversimplifying things and still consider where research has shown us that if you are a female, you are more likely to think, feel or behave in a certain way, though of course it doesn't mean that you definitely will. For example, we know that there's a height difference between the sexes: men are more likely to be taller than women. But we come across men all the time who are shorter than us, which doesn't negate the fact that men, on average, are taller than women. So, we're going to explore the nuances of how women tend to think and act and we can guarantee that it won't all apply to you if you're a female reader, while some of it may apply to you if you're a male reader. Understanding how our brains function, and how our social environments and experiences as women can impact the way our brains work, is hugely helpful in better understanding your relationship with sport and exercise, and in ensuring you get the best out of yourself in any arena of your life.

Emotion sensor

Just as we wish to banish the word 'hormonal' from being used to describe women's behaviour in the days before their period arrives, we'd also like to lose the label 'emotional'. The belief that women are more emotional than men has been called a 'master stereotype', meaning it is a widely held view that is pervasive across all of society.[4] The majority of men and women, old and young, from a range of cultural backgrounds, hold the belief that women are more emotional than men.[5]

The fact is, we are all emotional, just as we are all hormonal. Men don't have fewer emotions than women, but the way men and women perceive, process and respond to emotional stimuli tends to be different. As women, we are differently emotional, not more or less emotional. Women have a higher blood flow to brain regions that are responsible for verbal processing and emotion. This often means women express their emotions by externalizing and talking about them, compared with men, who often internalize emotions as a way of processing them. Increased blood flow to emotional brain regions such as the amygdala have been associated with higher levels of anxiety and mood symptoms in females, and may also explain why women are often more empathetic and intuitive than men.[6]

This idea that women are more empathetic than men has been supported by large-scale research assessing half a million people, concluding that the female brain is predominantly hard-wired for empathy, and that the male brain is predominantly hard-wired for understanding and building systems. The lead researcher of this work, Sir Simon Baron-Cohen, a clinical psychologist and professor of psychopathology, calls it the empathizing-systemizing (E-S) theory.[7] Being empathetic means you can identify another person's emotions and thoughts, and respond with appropriate emotion, intuitively figuring out how others feel. Systemizing means you analyse and explore how things work in order to understand the underlying 'rules' that control a system.

But what does this mean for active women? Sport is an emotional pursuit for everyone. But for women, research shows that sport can bring up specific emotional challenges such as body dissatisfaction, injury, bullying, eating disorders, coach conflicts, sexual abuse, performance expectations, self-criticism, social comparisons,[8] unequal or unfair treatment, and machismo and patronizing attitudes of male administrators, coaches and referees.[9] That's a whole heap of crap that potentially comes our way as active women, and it's been shown that women who have not developed the skills to deal with the demands they encounter in sport and exercise settings may experience negative outcomes such as poorer performance and high levels of distress. This may ultimately lead them to drop out of sport and exercise after being gradually ground down without the strategies to cope.[10] Those who stick it out and remain in their sport despite these negative influences often suffer mental and physical health issues as a result. Either way, it's not an ideal situation for women in sport and we all need to work together to change this culture.

Women tend to deal with emotions by talking about them; it's part of something called emotion-focused coping, where we actively do something to manage our emotional response to a stressful situation.[11] Our tendency, as women, to want to share emotions to help ourselves manage them can sometimes be at odds with the way men like to process or cope with stressors. Men tend to use problem-focused coping, where they try to 'fix' the situation itself. When a woman talks through how she feels about the fact that she hasn't been able to fit in any exercise this week, or that she didn't do as well in her 10k run as she wanted to, a male trainer or partner might go into problem-focused mode and try to fix the problem. If he doesn't think he knows how to fix it, he might feel frustrated by the expectation to try. But often, the woman doesn't want the problem fixed; she wants to process her emotions so that she can move on. This mismatch between how women communicate their emotions and how the men around them deal with that communication style is something we see all the time between female athletes and male coaches, and male PE teachers and female students. Men tell us it's one of the things they find most challenging when working with women, and vice versa.

It's completely normal for everyone to experience a range of emotions. Emotions are caused by our brain making sense of our bodily sensations and from our experiences of what's going on around us. In 2022, an Irish Football Association coach told the media that his female team had played poorly because, as women, they were more 'emotional' than male players.[12] The team had conceded a goal early in the match and it knocked their confidence, and with each new goal scored against them, their performance grew worse and worse. Of course these players were emotional. They wouldn't have been in the pitch if they weren't invested in being the best, in winning the match. Feeling emotions when the opposition scores, when you haven't played as well as you can, or when a teammate makes a poor play, is totally normal. It's what you do in response to it that can bring your performance down. The coach in this case would have been far better off trying to support his players to develop strategies to help them process that emotional response during that game. It's not a bad thing to be emotional in any given situation; the key is what you do with that emotion to achieve a positive end result.

In the heat of the moment, when a shot has been missed or a referee decision has gone against them, athletes use mental resetting techniques to process the surge of emotion that comes in that moment. Rather than letting it overcome them and impact the rest of their performance, the athletes have strategies to help reset their thinking. It's not just in the middle of a high-stakes sports match that these strategies can help; it's when your boss has made an unreasonable request, your kids have pushed your buttons, or the train that's taking you to your much-needed spin class gets cancelled. Mental resetting techniques are often 'doing' rather than 'thinking' strategies. Dr Jonathan Fader, a performance psychologist and author of *Life as Sport*, says it's really hard to 'think' yourself out of an emotional situation, so an action can often be much more effective for resetting.[13]

Mental resetting techniques include:

- **Deep breath in, deep breath out**
  This clears your mind and calms your nervous system. Even better than a single breath is 'box breathing', so called because a box has four sides: four seconds breathe in, four seconds hold, four seconds breathe out, four seconds hold. Repeat.[14]

- **Have a cue word that you say out loud, or a cue action**
  It could be a simple as saying 'move on' or 'protect your energy', or clicking your fingers, to redirect your brain out of the moment and remind you to let feelings pass.[15]

- **Adopt a winning posture**

  Have you heard of the power pose? Shared by Amy Cuddy in her TED Talk on body language, the idea is that a head-up, chest-out posture improves confidence in situations when you might need a boost, like before a big presentation. This posture can also work in moments of high emotion. It has been shown to reduce cortisol and improve tolerance for risk. It may also help reset from a negative experience.[16]

Selection day drama

We spoke to a top-level women's rugby team coach who had successfully coached both male and female teams about the main differences between them. He immediately started talking about team selection day. His experience with men's teams was that on selection day, he would individually sit down with each player for a couple of minutes and tell them whether they'd be playing at the weekend. Each player, regardless of whether or not they had been selected, would say, 'Yes, boss, thanks. See you on the training pitch.' Job done – back out to the pre-match training session. When the coach used the same strategy with women players, it didn't play out the same way. When a player was told she hadn't made the starting line-up, she showed her emotions about it. If she was upset, she needed time to be upset. She wanted to talk through the decision, understand why it had been made and know the reasons why someone else had made the line-up. The women players also cared about what had happened to their teammates. They were emotional not just about their own selection, but really cared and empathized with those around them who had or hadn't been selected. They needed to talk through the events with each other. Suddenly, the two minutes he'd set aside to deliver each player their selection news was nowhere near enough. His old method of running selection notification day did not work with the women he was now coaching. He persevered for a while, thinking the players would adapt to his approach, but all he got each week after the selection meeting was a group of unmotivated players who were angry with him, making that important pre-match practice a write-off.

This coach didn't need the research to tell him that women tend to process emotion differently to men, that they tend to be empathizers, recognizing and responding to the emotions of others, and that females tend to want to explore the rationale behind coaching decisions. These tendencies were self-evident, and the players knew what helped them accept and express their emotions in a helpful way. The players typically needed to take some time out, talk to friends, talk the process through with the coach and share how they felt, find a quiet space to rest and breathe, or have a walk around the pitch. To be an effective coach, he had to change the way he went about things with his women's team and recognize that they would play better if he gave them the time and space to process their emotions after the selection meeting. He began to set more time aside for selection conversations, where he could explain the reasons behind his decisions. He left enough time between selection conversations and pre-match training sessions for the players to process the information. Some players asked to receive the decision ahead of time, by text or email, so they could deal with their emotions before sitting down to talk with him. The outcome was entirely positive: the coach had a better relationship with his players, the players were happier and trained more effectively, and this led to the team achieving greater success.

You don't have to be a top-flight sportswoman for this to apply to you – we all experience the range of emotions those players felt on selection day. Find strategies that are helpful to you to process and express your emotions. Don't let emotions control you or impact your behaviour in a way you don't like.

Here are some tips that might help you process your emotions.

- **Get curious, but not too close**
  Be curious about your reaction to events as they happen: what feelings are these? Why did I react like that? What's happening? And then distance yourself a bit. Remind yourself that you are not your emotions. Use phrases like 'I notice I am feeling frustrated' rather than 'I'm frustrated' to keep space between you and your feelings.

- **Know what it feels like**
  What does your body do in response to events that spark your emotions – what does it feel like? Does your jaw clench, your stomach churn, or do you get tunnel vision? By paying attention to your body's signals when something is going on, you can tune in to heightened emotions, try resetting techniques and often stop yourself overthinking or spiralling downwards.

- **'Rumble' with your story**
  If you're thinking, 'I can't keep up with the pace, I'm not good enough', prod and poke at that feeling a bit. Ask yourself, 'What is actually true here? What story am I making up, and do I need to consider more information to make sense of my reaction?'

- **Address your basic needs**
  Hunger, thirst and being sedentary can interfere with how we process and express emotions. Do you need to eat, drink, get outside, move your body?

- **Breathe**

  Use the proven relaxation technique of box breathing. It's been used by US Navy Seals to come out of fight-or-flight mode so that they can calm down after combat.

- **Reframe**

  If you're feeling angry or disappointed by something, is there a way to reframe the situation? Say you can't make it to spin class because your partner is home late from work and they were going to look after the children. You're in your workout gear and have an hour to do something – how else can you move your body? A walk, a different class, find a workout video on YouTube? What did you learn from this that you can use for next time – is timing too tight to make the class? Does your partner need to set an alarm to remind them to leave work by a certain time?

- **Talk about it**

  Expressing emotion means that they don't pile up inside us like a debt that eventually becomes due. Taking thoughts out of your head and saying them out loud, either to yourself or to someone else, or writing them down, is a way of processing what you are feeling.

Tend and befriend

Let's talk about the time that science got it wrong when it came to describing how women cope with stress. In the 1930s, the fight-or-flight concept was coined to explain how our bodies and brains respond to threat or stress. You're probably familiar with the expression, meaning that when faced with a threatening situation, or in times of stress, our body prepares itself for action.

Our pupils dilate, our heart rate increases, more sugar is released into the bloodstream to give us instant energy and our body deprioritizes functions such as digestion to direct resources to our all-important muscles and brain. All of this happens courtesy of hormones, such as adrenaline and cortisol, sending signals throughout our body, allowing us to fight the threat or run like crazy away from it. This stress response has been, and still is, the accepted way we look at how humans respond in threatening situations. It's the one we were taught about in our medical and science degrees, and the one that comes up if you google 'the body's stress response'.

But early in the 2000s, a researcher called Shelley Taylor wasn't convinced that women *always* coped with stress with a fight or flight, based on her own experience. She began a series of experiments that looked at the biochemical and psychological responses to stress in women and found that women's responses were marked by a pattern of 'tend and befriend' rather than fight or flight. Tending involves nurturing activities designed to protect those closest to you, ones that promote safety and reduce distress, while befriending is developing social networks to ensure connected, collaborative action.[17]

First up: how did we simply not know about this for so long? It's that gender data gap again: prior to the mid-1990s, only about 17% of the participants in studies of biological responses to stress were women.[18] Thank goodness for Taylor and her crew of researchers at the University of California, Los Angeles (UCLA), whose work allowed us to discover that the fight-or-flight mechanism was probably at odds with both the biology of women and their role in early society. Women evolved as caregivers, so if a woman's response to stress was to fight, they risked leaving an infant behind if they lost. It's a lot more difficult to flee if you have to take a child along, too. Taylor and her colleagues realized that, instead of producing the fight-or-flight response in the face of threat, women are more likely to tend to their young and befriend others – specifically other women – in order to ensure their survival and the survival of their genes.

The research shows that women have a whole neurochemistry and neurocircuitry that is different from men's and that supports this tend-and-befriend model of stress response. For example, women naturally have more oxytocin than men. Oxytocin is essential for childbirth, breastfeeding and strong parent–child bonding, but the hormone can also help promote trust, empathy and social connection. In experiments where female animals are given an injection of oxytocin, they behave as if a social switch has been turned on, seeking out more social contact with their friends and relatives. Oestrogen may also play a role in the tend-and-befriend response, since it amplifies the relaxing effect of oxytocin, making it even more effective.

What the UCLA researchers spent many years unpicking and proving, most women will have had a hunch about long before reading it here. Using the support of our friends and family to help us manage stress, process emotion, and generally deal with life, is what women have been doing well for centuries. Even the name the three of us use, The Well HQ, came about partly because the well was one of the first meeting places for women. Young women typically had the daily chore of collecting water from the well, and it became a place where they could meet, talk, befriend and support one another. Fast forward to the present day, and while the well might now be a bottle of prosecco, a flat white or a group run, women still reap the benefits of a social support system when it comes to coping with the stresses and strains of everyday life.

Coping with stress by seeking out social support and nurturing others is as vital to our health and well-being as the food we eat, how much sleep we get, and how much we exercise. Research shows that ties with family and close friends are beneficial to our physical health, while social isolation increases the risk for *all* causes of death, including heart disease, cancer, stroke, accidents or suicide.[19] And women don't need to keep the benefits to themselves. Despite all the evolutionary and biological evidence pointing to the fact that women display the tend-and-befriend response more, men can also adopt this response.

We no longer have to face the kind of vicious predators our ancestors did; the stressors we encounter are less life-threatening in the short term, but they are much more likely to keep us in a state of chronic stress, as one follows another in quick succession. In order to benefit from the tend-and-befriend approach, you don't even have to look at it as a male–female mindset but see social connections of support and collaboration as a really effective strategy that helps all humans cope with stress.

In confidence

In all walks of life, success, it turns out, correlates just as closely with our self-confidence as it does with how good we actually are. In school, college, business and sport, women are consistently reported as having less confidence than men.[20] We are constantly told this is what holds us back. But research from Meghan Huntoon at Northern Illinois University suggests that it's not that women lack confidence in their skills, competence or ideas, but instead that they are reluctant to shout about it, for fear of the social consequences of asserting or promoting themselves.[21] Is it possible that self-confidence doesn't differ between the sexes, but the consequences of appearing self-confident does? Surely the solution needs to be to challenge the double standard in workplaces, support women's ability to promote their own achievements without backlash, get people to recognize their biases about confident women and hold men to a higher standard of compassionate behaviour.[22]

Do these findings transfer to our active pursuits as well as our professional ones? In sport, confidence is more helpful than harmful; indeed, self-confidence is an essential skill for athletic success.[23] Demonstrating visible self-belief gives you a distinct advantage in sport. It can inflate others' perception of your competence, leading them to believe you've got what it takes to win – regardless of whether you have or not – and giving you an edge. However, the idea that women don't choose to show confidence outwardly, despite having it inwardly, persists in sport. Research has shown that men are much more likely to confidently state a big goal, such as 'I'm going to run the London Marathon next year', whereas women are not comfortable vocalizing such an ambitious target.[24] Despite being equally sure that they can achieve a big goal, women might not focus on the goal itself but gain confidence from attending to all the important elements of the training and preparation necessary to help them achieve it. There's no right or wrong approach; what's important is to use strategies that work for you, and for the narrative around confidence not to rely so heavily on the outward expression of self-belief, but to acknowledge that being 'quietly confident' is a strength too.

There is a difference in how sportswomen and -men derive their confidence, though, and it's important to be aware of this because if you, and those who support you, can tune in to what it takes to make you feel like a champion, then it's likely to pay off in better performance. Research shows that women derive confidence less from their coach or personal trainer's encouragement and positive feedback, and much more from mastering skills and achieving personal goals, as opposed to men, who tend to derive confidence from comparing themselves with others and winning.[25]

Women also derive confidence and motivation from the quality of the relationship with the person training, coaching or teaching them. Whereas men tend to draw confidence from the quality of their trainer or coach – i.e. how successful that person is and how well the people or teams they have coached have performed – women want a coach or trainer who is interested in them as a person, more broadly than just their sports performance or fitness regime; someone who cares about and is interested in them, and understands what's going on in their life.[26]

We see this all the time at The Well HQ: a fitness trainer whose classes are rammed every week because she gets to know everyone there and knows what's on their plate at the moment, making those that attend her classes feel a connection to her that keeps them coming back; the netball coach who has a session every week where the team get to learn something about the culture from each of the players – an opportunity to share something important beyond their netball; the PE teacher who takes time to get to know a bunch of girls who have stopped showing up to sports, so he or she can put on activities that better connect to their interests. Knowing what builds our confidence and our motivation to stay engaged with sport or exercise is so important, because it's one thing getting up off the sofa once to choose to exercise, but to keep on doing it, you need an environment that draws you back.

The big P

Perfectionism is a self-destructive and addictive belief system that says, 'I am what I accomplish and how well I accomplish it.' Perfectionism is a fear of shame, judgement and blame, and of disappointing others. In her book *The Gifts of Imperfection*, Brené Brown likens perfectionism to a suit of armour that we trudge around in, assuming it will protect us, whereas in actual fact it's the thing that's weighing us down and stopping us realizing our full potential.[27] Research shows that perfectionism hampers success. In fact, it's often the path to depression, anxiety, addiction and life paralysis.[28]

Studies show that women are more likely to exhibit perfectionist tendencies than men, and, interestingly, perfectionism is increasing over time, with recent generations of young people demanding more of themselves and others than ever before.[29] It's not that striving to be your best or improving yourself are bad traits – they are some of the best ones of all. But overdone, they can fall into the realms of perfectionism, because perfectionism is not about healthy achievements and personal growth; it's the belief that this next challenge, this next race, this next goal, can define us, our pursuit of it can cocoon us, and achieving it will make others proud and happy. Healthy striving is self-focused: 'How can I improve?' Perfectionism is other-focused: 'What will they think?'

Yet perfectionism is an unattainable goal. There is simply no such thing as perfect. In the pursuit of sporting goals, perfectionism can be compulsive and debilitating. Success in sport is built on achievement, on being judged on your last performance, how fit you currently are or what your body looks like. If you're not performing well, if you don't make the team, even if you don't look as 'good' in your workout gear as the instructor does, then the perfectionist deep inside might tell you that you need to be different, you need to 'improve', you need to change to be worthy of recognition or of belonging in your sport, your club or your gym. In contrast to this, healthy-striving self-talk is about acknowledging your imperfections in an honest and compassionate way, without shame or the fear that finds you wanting in the eyes of others. It's about recognizing that you're worthy of belonging here in sport or fitness, regardless of what your 5km time says, what brand of bike you ride, or how much you weigh. If you want to change those things, do them for you, for your health, for your enjoyment, your sense of accomplishment or inspiration. Don't do them because you think they define you.

Baz

I have worked with many perfectionists over my years as a pelvic floor coach and I know first-hand how disastrous it can be as an approach to sustainable health and fitness behaviour. Of course, I want every woman to do her pelvic floor exercises every day, and when women start working with me that's exactly what they do: they crack on and get the work done. But if they have a perfectionist, all-or-nothing mindset, and for whatever reason they miss a day, they tumble into a downward spiral of negative self-talk about how rubbish they are at doing exercises and they give up completely. That's them done, until they see me again for a pep talk and a reset. This roller coaster of doing everything perfectly or not doing it at all doesn't serve us well, which is why I introduced my 'low bar' concept. The low bar is what you feel you can do every day regardless of what life may throw at you. It's irrelevant where you set this bar; you just need to be confident that you can do it. It's a two-out-of-ten effort. It may be 'I'll eat breakfast by 8 a.m. and do one pelvic floor exercise or walk 3,000 steps today' – whatever. It won't get you 'big results' but what it does is keep you progressing with your fitness, even at a snail's pace, and stop the downward spiral and negative self-talk that occurs when you give up completely. This is a really useful concept within the context of health, fitness and participation. It helps women to adopt a compassionate approach to themselves, which serves them much better in the long run.

The sport and fitness industry can make us feel rubbish if we don't live up to our own expectations, those of others or those set by the warped reality we see through Instagram filters. How can we arm ourselves with the psychological skills that help us thrive as active women? For that, we need vulnerability and self-compassion.[30]

Brené Brown defines vulnerability as uncertainty, risk and emotional exposure. Vulnerability is not winning or losing, it's having the courage to show up when the outcome is uncertain, about being seen for who you truly are and to ask for what you truly need. As an active woman, every time you stand on the starting line of a parkrun or turn up to gym glass or the local pool, you show vulnerability, you open yourself up to the possibility that you might be judged, criticized or not do as well as you or anyone else expects, but you get stuck in anyway. And that's where sport has historically judged vulnerability as a weakness, as showing your flaws, letting your competition see your weak spots, being meek, accepting failure or not being aggressive enough.[31] In fact, a 2019 research paper posed the question 'Is there an upside to vulnerability in sport?', implying that, up until then, individuals in sport were less likely or unwilling to show vulnerability because they anticipated being perceived as weak or treated unfairly.[32]

Baz

I was always on the very edge of being in the boat. I rowed in the GB women's eight, and the first seven seats were always filled before I got a look in. I was desperate to get that final seat in one of the most successful teams in the world. To do so, there was no way I was going to show weakness or vulnerability. I did all I could to hide anything that could jeopardize my selection, which meant hiding my emotion, my pain, my fear of failure and certainly everything female about me. I couldn't be my whole, true self. This meant that I didn't ask for help when I needed it – like when I lost my periods or wasn't coping. I didn't know how to be vulnerable in sport without it affecting my chances of success, because the system I was operating within saw vulnerability as weakness.

Yet researchers from the Swedish School of Sport and Health Sciences and the University of Portsmouth recognized how useful vulnerability can be in athletes and coaches alike.[33] They found that having the courage and capacity to share experiences and shortcomings, and to seek support – knowing when to share, with whom, and to what extent – is a psychological strength in sport.

Bella

Vulnerability is an essential tool for being a doctor. Just as in sport, people often wonder how that works in my profession. No one wants to sit in my clinic and hear me say, 'I don't know' or, 'I feel really out of my depth here because I've never seen a case like this before.' But that's not what vulnerability means to me. For me, it's saying, 'I don't know the best way forward here because this is not my area of expertise and I need to contact someone who does know the answer, because I want to make sure I give you the most up-to-date and correct information on this.' I admit to not knowing, and I don't make excuses or flannel my way through the appointment. My job is about building trust and pretending to know it all doesn't cultivate trust. Then, at the end of the day, I share my feelings of not knowing with a colleague, reflect on the outcome and ultimately learn from the experience. Knowing that I can have an honest conversation about what turns out to be a common experience in my profession, means that I don't carry around feelings of frustration, guilt or shame. It helps me be resilient in what is often a very demanding job.

If we acknowledge that sport and fitness are arenas often filled with self-judgement and perfectionism, we also have to accept that these tendencies limit our ability to be courageous, vulnerable and to take risks, and that isn't a good recipe for those of us who want to pursue dreams of being fitter, healthier or performing better. However, research shows that self-compassion, giving yourself a break, and being gentle with yourself during difficult moments, can help you develop a strong foundation from which you can reach for the things that really matter to you – the things that require you to risk, to take bold, courageous action, and to let yourself be seen by others.

Kristin Neff leads the self-compassion research lab at the University of Texas at Austin, where she studies how we can develop this essential skill.[34] And it really is a skill: it can be learned, and it improves and gets easier with practice. Better still, compassion is like a virus – it spreads quickly – but with much nicer outcomes. When we are self-compassionate, others around us feel free to be compassionate too, and that creates stronger and more authentic connections between us.

What is self-compassion, apart from being kind to yourself when you've mucked up or fallen short? Self-compassion has three elements:

- **Self-kindness**
  Being warm and understanding to ourselves when we suffer, fail or feel inadequate, rather than ignoring our pain or flagellating ourselves with self-criticism. Talking to ourselves, like we would talk to a good friend who was suffering.

- **Common humanity**

  Recognizing that suffering and feelings of inadequacy are part of the shared human experience – something we all go through, rather than something that happens to oneself alone.

- **Mindfulness**

  Taking a balanced approach to negative emotion so that our feelings are neither suppressed nor exaggerated. We cannot ignore our pain and feel compassion for it at the same time. Mindfulness requires that we don't over-identify with thoughts and feelings; that we don't overthink them and get swept away by negativity.[35]

Amber Mosewich, of the University of British Columbia, has taken the study of self-compassion into sport, in particular into women's sport, as a mindset tool to allow athletes to reach their full potential in an adaptive, healthy way (as opposed to mal-adaptive strategies such as addition, numbing and avoidance). The reason Mosewich believes self-compassion is an important tool for active women is that women generally have lower self-compassion and greater tendency towards rumination, compared with men.[36] This rumination and self-criticism causes problems in coping with stress, challenging situations and failure, which in turn has the potential to wreak havoc across active women's whole lives – from our motivation to exercise, to what we eat, to how confident we are. Research also shows that self-compassion can be particularly useful for younger women and girls dealing with low body confidence, low self-esteem or dysfunctional body image, tendencies that we know are prevalent in active women and that can be overwhelming during teenage years. In her research, Mosewich found self-compassion practices to be effective in helping active women manage self-criticism, rumination and concern over mistakes. She concluded that fostering a self-compassionate frame of mind is a potential coping resource for women athletes dealing with stress and challenge in sport.[37]

As part of her research, she asked active women to complete a short exercise for seven days.[38] Each day they were asked to think about a negative event in their training, workout or sport that had occurred over the past week and to provide a description of the event, including what happened leading up to the event, who was there, what happened, and any thoughts and actions that happened during the event. Then, they were asked to use journaling (a fancy name for writing stuff down each day) to do the following.

1. List ways in which other people experience similar events.
2. Write a paragraph expressing understanding, kindness and concern to themselves (to help them with this, because we are often much harder on ourselves than we would be on others, the women were asked to write as if you were talking to a close friend having a similar struggle).
3. Describe the event in an objective and unemotional manner – this was meant to allow them to recognize and acknowledge it, without overthinking it.

Journaling in this way regularly (and you don't have to do it every day of the week, but more frequently is better at first) is an effective way to start developing more self-compassion in your life; a way to develop more vulnerability and courage. Over time, you won't always need to write it down, but run through these steps in your mind.

Baz

Jemima is an impressive woman, and a colleague and friend of us at The Well HQ. She's also a keen runner, having made the move in her late forties from recreational runner to serious PB pursuer. She trains hard, and she has fierce ambitions to set a sub-three-hour marathon time. But recently, after a ten-mile race didn't go to plan, her Instagram story struck us as a perfect lesson in vulnerability and compassion in an active woman. First, she posted a time that she was disappointed with on social media. Not for 'Oh no, you're great really'-type support, but to share a common human experience, one that us active folk know too well. You feel ready for it, you feel fit for it, and then halfway around, your body says 'not today' and your performance falls short of your expectations. She said she was disappointed, she told us about her planned minute-per-mile pace and how far behind she fell as the race went on.

She said she had felt gloomy all day, so she checked her time for a ten-mile race a decade ago. It was thirteen minutes – twenty-five seconds slower than her current time. She balanced her gloominess with gratitude and happiness that, at nearly fifty, she was smashing her nearly forty-year-old self! She rounded off her post with the words 'Good to be disappointed. Good to be kind to yourself. Good to want to give it another go.' In that short post she showed self-kindness, humility and mindfulness, and it gave her the resilience to dust herself off and move forward with a positive mindset. A few weeks later, Jemima was the first woman home in a sixteen-mile race.

As you can imagine, becoming self-compassionate doesn't happen overnight and just because someone told you that it was a helpful thing to be if you wanted a happier, less stressful life. As with any new skill or way of thinking, you have to believe it to be valuable, you have to practise it and you must have the motivation and patience to keep practising until it becomes more automatic.

Broken brains

Our brains are precious. Despite the fact that they overthink and overwhelm us sometimes, they're amazing: they're made up of one hundred billion neurons, which send signals around our brain and into our body at speeds of over 260 miles per hour. But there's an alarming gender gap when it comes to keeping our brains safe.

Research shows that women and girls may be more susceptible to sport-related concussions than men; and that not only are their symptoms more prolonged compared with men's, the time it takes them to fully return to sport is longer, too.[39] The gender gap comes because we aren't translating this research into practice – there are no sex-specific guidelines for concussion; there are no school, work or sport protocols, or educational resources, for women who suffer concussion; and sport, academic, military and medical communities do not have any female-specific guidelines about concussion. The most recent consensus-statement from the Concussion in Sport Group on how to diagnose and rehabilitate sport concussion failed to identify women as a population at greater risk of concussion, despite raising the point that 'special' populations should be managed differently.[40] They made recommendations for elite and young athletes, and did briefly mention that girls might be at increased risk compared with boys, but the guidelines – which are endorsed by national governing bodies of many sports – do not yet consider the specific prevalence, diagnosis and treatment in females.

Professor Tracey Covassin is a leading researcher in concussion. Inspired to work in this field by her love of ice hockey, the Canadian academic noticed that most of the sports concussion research was being done in ice hockey and American football, and exclusively on men. When she looked at what we know about brain injury in sport in females, she saw the prevalence of sport-related concussion in women was twice as high than in men, and her journey to understanding why began.[41]

In general, sport doesn't have a great track record of taking action on the issue of concussion and in 2021, UK MPs released a report that expressed grave concerns about how concussion was dealt with in sport. In elite sport, they said, athletes had put their future health on the line in the interests of achieving sporting success for their country, and in grassroots sport with mass participation, they found what they described as 'negligible' efforts to track brain injuries and monitor long-term impacts.[42] But these findings were for everyone yet based only on data from men's sport. There's an urgent need to investigate the best ways to protect the brains of girls and women in sport, too.

What's more alarming is recent research which has identified that it's not just concussions which could be causing harm to our long-term brain health, but 'sub-concussions' too. Simply put, concussions are the hits to the brain that cause symptoms. Concussions have symptoms because the brain is shaken violently enough that brain cells are damaged to the point where they don't work properly. Sub-concussive impacts are those that are below that concussion threshold: the brain is shaken, but not so violently that brain cells are damaged enough to experience symptoms. Sub-concussions can happen hundreds of times during, for example, football, rugby or hockey matches. Bodies colliding, tackling, falling to the ground and heading the ball, all cause sub-concussive impact to the brain.[43]

In her 2022 TED talk, Dr Emer MacSweeney warns that it is these sub-concussions during sport which, over time, cause an accumulation of microtrauma to the brain and can lead to the development of Chronic Traumatic Encephalopathy (CTE).[44] Signs and symptoms of CTE include difficulties with thinking and emotions, mental health issues and early onset neurodegenerative disease such as Alzheimer's and dementia. There is no cure for CTE and Dr MacSweeney describes it as a 'silent killer in contact sports'. She also warns that hardly any women's brains are included in the research of CTE, yet with the rise of female participation in contact sports, and the greater prevalence of neurodegenerative disease in women – who make up two thirds of all dementia patients – there is an urgent need to understand brain injury in sport from a female perspective.[45]

In a 2020 study of 80,000 athletes in American high schools, researchers found that girls were twice as likely to suffer a concussion, yet it was boys who were more likely to be taken off the field of play after a concussion. We aren't being vigilant enough about girls and women suffering concussion, and we're not recognizing that females might need different treatment and rehabilitation protocols. The reasons why this sex difference exists is still poorly understood, and more research in this area is vital. However, what we know so far is that physical differences in women – such as having smaller heads and less neck strength – means they have greater head acceleration, which is what causes concussion.[46] A heavy head on a strong neck, as in males, can withstand a lot more force before the acceleration is so great that it causes damage to the brain.

Interestingly, the hormones of the menstrual cycle may also play a role in our experience of concussion.[47] There is some research that looked at a large number of women reporting to hospital with concussion and found that those experiencing concussion in the second half of the cycle, when progesterone is high, experienced poorer outcomes a month later.[48] Rather than progesterone being the bad guy, these researchers think that because progesterone has neuroprotective qualities, when women are injured during this phase of the cycle, the stress of the concussion causes progesterone to suddenly fall, and there is some kind of withdrawal effect from the progesterone that impacts our recovery. These findings suggest that at best a blood test, or at least a question about the date of a woman's last period to identify where she is in her cycle, might be important things for medical practitioners to think about when a woman presents with concussion. Knowing that a woman is in a high-progesterone phase of her cycle might indicate that she is at risk of poorer long-term outcomes and that she may need more vigilant monitoring or return-to-play support. Until we have more research in this area, we won't know if recommendations like this could really help improve the care of women with brain injuries.

Although research has been ongoing for nearly two decades, we still don't know enough about the potential causes of the difference in concussion between the sexes despite having these hypotheses about neck strength, brain anatomy and hormones. It's almost certain that the different explanations aren't mutually exclusive and, like any other injury, it may happen only when some of the risk factors combine to create the perfect storm. What's also concerning are the long-term consequences of concussion. When retired athletes started to be diagnosed with dementia – including footballing legends Bobby Charlton and Nobby Stiles, both part of England's 1966 winning World Cup team, who were diagnosed with dementia in their eighties and seventies respectively, and also Welsh rugby player Ryan Jones and his British Lions teammate Steve Thompson, who were diagnosed in their forties – it sparked widespread calls to fund more research and spread more awareness about the link between playing sport and neurodegeneration later in life.

We hope that the research will carefully explore the long-term risks in both men *and* women. Since we know concussion is more prevalent in women, and manifests with different symptoms, we could hypothesize that women are at greater risk of long-term consequences, too. The hypothesis is strengthened when we consider that after menopause, women's risk of dementia is believed to increase due to a drop in oestrogen levels when a woman enters her post-menopausal years, and oestrogen protects brain cells from damage and prevents them from degenerating. So, once again, hormones might become another risk factor in this type of injury and its long-term effects. Let's hope the funders and researchers of these exciting studies into the links between concussion and neurodegenerative diseases don't fall foul of the gender data gap and that the research serves to understand concussion in both men and women, separately and equally.

But while we wait for more research, what else can we do to protect the brains of girls and women in sport? Dr Elisabeth Williams from Swansea University researches concussion in women's rugby, and suggests that one of the most important things we can do is include training that develops neck strength.[49] Women have less neck strength than men due to their smaller total neck muscle volume, meaning that when they fall, their head is more likely to hit the ground than men who have a greater ability to hold their head away from direct contact. Teaching girls how to fall safely would be a good move. There's also a myth that skull caps and helmets protect our brains when we play rugby, ride bikes or horses. In fact, while these helmets protect our skulls from being damaged, they do nothing to stop the forces which act on the brain and cause it to become damaged inside of our skull. There is now a headband available which is the first product of its kind to offer brain (rather than skull) protection in sport.[50] Dr Mac-Sweeney suggests that everyone who participates in sports which involve contact or the risk of falls should be wearing such brain protection to reduce the risk of developing CTE. Mouthguards have also been developed with built-in accelerometers to provide data on the forces acting on the head, which means we don't have to rely on symptoms to tell us whether the brain has undergone trauma during sport. Applying approaches from other sports to reduce potential injury could also help: in youth baseball there are limits on how many pitches can be made by one person, because research shows that this prevents injury and long-term damage to the elbow.[51] Maybe we could get to the point where information from technology worn by the players will allow us to limit how much brain impact can be experienced before a player is removed from the field of play, or a certain number of days of enforced recovery is mandated. There's no doubt that something needs to change to make contact sport safe for everyone, and to protect our lifelong brain and mental health.

How to be mentally well

- Acknowledge that while there's no such thing as a male or female brain, the influence of our biology, and our experiences, often makes women and men think and behave differently. Understanding this will help us create environments and relationships where everyone gets what they need.
- Build strong connections with your colleagues, teachers, coaches and trainers since women tend to gain motivation through the strength in their relationships.
- Accept that women take time to process decisions and want to talk about it – go with it, don't fight it.
- Recognize that being emotional is not a weakness. Developing strategies to process emotion can help us avoid getting stuck on a doomed thought-spiral.
- Be prepared to show vulnerability. While this can be particularly hard in the sporting arena, which has a tendency towards judgement and secrecy, psychological safety is compatible with high performance – we can feel nurtured and supported, and still pursue ambitious goals.
- Dismantle perfectionism and build up self-compassion to help cope with the inevitable stresses and challenges in sport and in life.
- Learn how to recognize the signs and symptoms of concussion and what to do if it happens to you or to those around you, particularly if you do sport, or you support girls in sport.
- Explore strategies to reduce concussion and sub-concussion risk – including training for neck strength or wearing brain protection.

Chapter 11

Well Women, Across Our Lives

Across a woman's life, her body will go through significant changes that will affect how she feels physically and emotionally, from starting periods in her teens, developing breasts and growing into different shapes, to going through perimenopause and into menopause. These are not illnesses or crises, injuries or emergencies, but normal and natural transitions from one stage of life to another.

Thank goodness a 'Stop moving' sign is no longer put on women going through these transitions! Yet we are still woefully uneducated at each of these life stages about what's going on with our body, and particularly uncatered for when it comes to being and staying active or sporty during these times.[1] In this chapter we explore the two inevitable life stages a female will experience, puberty and menopause, and how these may impact on our ability to be active, and how being active impacts our lives. We haven't included the pre- and post-natal stages in this book, although we acknowledge that pregnancy, childbirth and the post-natal life phases are really important times in a woman's life, albeit they are not experienced by all women, through choice or circumstance.

Don't be the ostrich that buries her head in the sand and has a strategy of just ignoring everything in the belief that it will pass. Unfortunately, our bodies don't work like that. Just because you exercise every day or can run really fast or are on an elite team, this doesn't give you any points to trade for an easy, symptom-free cruise through puberty or menopause. Wouldn't it be amazing if that were the case? Instead, the best tools in your toolbox are knowledge and the confidence to use it, which is what this chapter is all about.

Girls moving and thriving through puberty

The changes happening inside a girl's body during puberty have some pretty significant effects on how she feels emotionally and physically, and alter the appearance of her body. That's just the biology part. The societal dynamics and pressures around being a young woman are also complex, and about 90% of the time, girls' anxiety levels are greater than they need to be.[2] During teenage years, girls can wake up anxious every day. They check their phone and social media, sometimes comparing themselves to other girls' Instagrammable lives. They worry about acne or the appearance of a new, shapelier figure; they worry about what they're eating and whether it will make them gain weight. They worry about not getting good grades or not fitting in at school. If they're active or sporty, they worry about how to manage periods during sport, they can be embarrassed around newly developed breasts showing through sports kit, or worry about what they look like when they get hot and sweaty.

Being active and going through puberty is a pretty tough combination. At a time when you don't recognize your body – what it looks and feels like – you are expected to move it and, in sport, have its performance scrutinized, measured and judged. So it's no wonder that by the end of puberty, 64% of girls will have dropped out of sport altogether – disengaging with physical activity at over twice the rate of boys.[3] And while the reasons for this drop-out from sport and exercise in girls are wide-ranging – from lack of confidence, not enough choice of activities, sport being seen as unfeminine, being academic prioritized over being active, lack of access or parental support – there is no doubt that falling out of love with moving our bodies in adolescence coincides with falling out of love with our bodies full stop.

Sadly, the education that girls (and boys) get at school about their bodies and puberty, and being physically active during puberty, is sparse. There has been some improvement in the UK over the past decade, but the few lessons that girls get focus on the mechanics of ovaries and fallopian tubes, uteruses and vaginas, and then a kind of 'damage control' – don't get pregnant and don't get an STD. What's missing is often the link between biology and behaviour – the effect that our ovaries and the hormones they produce have on our emotions and how we experience the world. They certainly miss the mark when it comes to talking to girls about their changing body in the context of sport and exercise. These lessons, particularly with younger girls, don't have to be about sex and babies; they can be about body literacy, learning about how your hormones can affect you physically and emotionally, how to track your menstrual cycle and how to manage periods when you want to be active, or how breasts will eventually develop and need supporting with a sports bra when you exercise.

In a study by the University of Portsmouth Research Group in Breast Health, 87% of teens reported an issue related to their breasts (such as pain, movement, bra fit, embarrassment) that was a barrier to doing exercise.[4] The study evaluated the impact of delivering an hour of education to girls about breast development, and breasts and exercise. After the education session, girls reported feeling less embarrassed about their breasts, more confident about choosing the right bra, and a desire to do more exercise as a result. Education can be so powerful at this age, but only if it's delivered on the right topics, in the right way, by the right people (and not the teacher who drew the short straw that term!). And we know that saying more education is needed is much easier than actually getting more education into an already overstretched school system, but it's not impossible. In 2022, the outcomes of a public consultation by the UK government identified that it was imperative to 'improve the quality and accessibility of information and education of women's health'.[5] We hope that future generations of girls are empowered by more and better education about their bodies as more investment and infrastructure is given to women's health education.

But it's not just schools that are responsible for sharing the knowledge. Parents play an important part, because their biases and beliefs are so influential on their children's attitudes to their bodies during adolescence. Experts emphasize that attitudes of parents are particularly important in determining how girls cope with their changing bodies. In her book about the impact of hormones on the brain, Sarah McKay suggests that if we don't treat puberty as a crisis or project our own negative experiences on to girls, they'll be much more likely to thrive.[6] Equally, research shows that when a girl's first period is acknowledged positively or celebrated as a rite of passage, instead of being ignored or expressed as negative, they are more likely to have positive body image and engage in health behaviours that support good sexual and reproductive health.

What's happening inside?

Puberty can begin in a girl's body as early as eight or nine years old, or as late as sixteen. Every woman is different and often girls follow in their mothers' footsteps in terms of things like the age they start their periods. Knowing that girls as young as eight may be about to start their journey through puberty means that, as parents or teachers of young girls, we need to start having conversations with them about puberty, and what changes the body will go through, from an early age. We have delivered talks on the menstrual cycle to classes of nine-year-olds and, when given some information and an open floor for questions, they asked some of the best questions and sparked the liveliest discussions we've had! From asking whether the blood 'spurts' out or what happens if you put in two tampons, to whether you can die from bleeding during a period, young girls have a curiosity about puberty not yet marred by being in the depths of it. Baz has even taught this age group about how to do their pelvic floor exercises. With the right tone and level of detail, we have only had positive experiences as girls get to grips with why it's important to know about their body, and how awesome it is.

Breasts are one of the first things to develop during puberty, and the appearance of breast buds usually indicates that periods will start within two years. Periods don't usually arrive without warning signs across the rest of the body, so we can use those cues, such as changes in the breasts, appearance of pubic hair, and growth of feet and then body size, to start having really positive and informative discussions with girls about what's next on the horizon for them.

One of the things that girls can struggle with, especially if they are active, is the changing shape of their body. The hormones that arrive during puberty tell a female body to lay down fat cells around the hips and bottom, as well as to develop breast tissue. This gives girls a curvier figure and changes the way they look and feel. In boys, male sex hormones can often improve athletic performance, strength and power, but for active girls there may be a temporary plateau in how well they perform in their chosen sport and they may experience a decline in body control. This may be most noticeable in sports that require good balance, such as gymnastics, or skill-based sports such as team games or racket sports.

The important thing to remember is that this is a transition phase of a girl's life – what her body looks and feels like during her teenage years, and how it performs, will not necessarily be linearly related to how it will look, feel and perform later on. What's important, if you are a parent of, or working with, very active and sporty girls, is to stay supportive, be patient and consistent with training, ensure they are well-fuelled and full of energy, and don't let anyone constantly put down or chastise them about their body and how it's working during this vulnerable time.

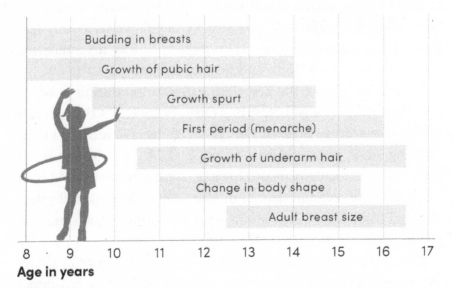

Puberty timeline in girls

Take some of the stress out of starting

The trouble with starting and having periods in the teenage years is that they are unpredictable. Teenagers don't yet know what their body feels like in the days leading up to their period, and cycles in the first two years of having periods can be really variable in length. Periods start when girls least expect them, and they can be heavier in some months than others. That's why we always encourage parents and teachers to have 'caught short' kits anywhere girls might be, kept in the toilets, in their school bags, and in kit bags when you travel away for matches. And what's most important is to ensure that girls know the products are there – have the conversation about where the products are and that girls are welcome to help themselves any time they need to. Lots of people already take the important step of making sure they always have period products for any girls who need them, but they forget to tell the girls where they are, which means they still have to ask the awkward 'Does anyone have a spare product?' question when they realize they've come on unexpectedly.

It's common for girls to be somewhere outside the home, and away from parents, when they get their first period. This is particularly true for sporty girls, who will probably spend more time away from home, at training before or after school, or at matches or competitions at the weekend, plus residential training camps, tours or even competitions abroad. That's why it's so important that girls know about periods before their first one arrives. Tell girls honestly about periods: what happens (blood comes out of the vagina for a few days every month or so) and how (it kind of trickles out, and you can't stop and start it like you do a wee), and what we do about it (we use period products that collect the blood so it doesn't leak out of our pants), and show them how products are used (but don't get them to try putting in a tampon when they are not bleeding – it's really painful to remove a tampon that's still dry).

We often get asked if it's OK for girls to wear a tampon when they first start having periods, particularly for active girls who would benefit from the choice of wearing a tampon during sport. The answer is that you can use tampons from your very first period if you want – they are totally safe, as long as you know how often to change them and you find the right size and absorbency so they can be comfortably inserted and removed. The biggest barrier we find with girls and tampons is not knowing how to insert them. We find that girls need quite a lot of encouragement to look at their vulva and vagina with a mirror, or explore it with their fingers so they know exactly what's down there and where the tampon goes. But by doing this, we can become much more comfortable and confident about all the bits of our body.

It's tough to talk

We totally understand that having these conversations about puberty, about bodies and what's happening to them, can be tricky. And we know it's perhaps a teenager's least favourite thing to talk about to parents or teachers. But we do need to talk to our girls.

Emma

I know how tough this audience can be! I've toured the country talking at many schools, to sports scholars and whole year groups, and at the beginning it felt like my toughest gig. When girls' periods first start, they are irregular, and the symptoms can be more severe than they will ultimately end up being years later. When I speak to groups of teenage athletes, there is definitely a different mindset around what they think of their body and how willing they are to better understand it, compared with, say, athletes in their early twenties. As women mature, they settle into their body, with breasts, a different body shape, and a monthly bleed, and they're really excited to know more about how it works, how they can tune in to it and how they can use this to optimize sport or enjoyment of exercise. During puberty, however, girls aren't always so keen. I've sat in front of many groups of teenage girls, all red-faced and crossed arms, knowing that each of them is wondering why the person in front of them is getting so excited about their amazing body, when they don't feel the same way. That's OK: just putting the information out there and introducing the idea that, as a woman, you can be in the driving seat of your cycle, rather than being at the mercy of it, and that it can help as well as hinder performance, and that your body is something to be celebrated, will plant some very empowering seeds.

Not even over the starting line

Unfortunately, a common (but not normal) conversation we have with parents of very sporty girls begins with 'My daughter is seventeen and hasn't started her period yet – should I be worried?' It's really important to be aware that a young woman hasn't started her periods by the time she's sixteen, and to support her to discuss this with a doctor. Dr Bella has this conversation regularly in her surgery, and will go through a family history – such as asking when the mother started periods, which may be relevant – and find out whether there are concerns around exercise and eating that may need further investigations, such as an examination, blood tests or scans.

It might be nothing, and normal for her particular body, but in very sporty girls it can be a sign that they aren't getting the balance of training, recovery and nutrition right and are suffering from RED-S, as previously explained. Girls need to know (and be proud of the fact) that their periods are a vital sign of health, and that not having periods can be down to experiencing energy deficiency, whether that's not starting periods, or starting but then losing them. Energy deficit can simply be caused by the fact that teenagers just aren't very good at getting their diets right, especially if they're doing lots of training. They might not have time between school and after-school activities, or they might not know what's healthy, nutritious fuel for their activity, or they might just underestimate how much energy their school/sport/social lifestyle requires.

Body image

Sometimes girls get their eating wrong on purpose, and consciously restrict the type and amount of food they eat to be slim. Body image is especially an issue for girls in sport. As they look to other girls and women who are having success, and try to emulate them, if they see lean and light older athletes doing well, they will associate lighter bodyweights and slimness with success, with little regard for the fact that losing weight quickly, not eating enough, or not fuelling with the right type of food at the right time, will have far greater negative consequences on their performance. This is also a time when the choice of language used is critical. Saying, or even implying, that a girl looks 'big' or 'fat' can be the point at which a sporty girl's journey forks, pointing them down a road that far too often ends in physical or mental illness, or in injury.

Young women are an at-risk population for eating disorders; eating disorders can present at any age, but the peak age presentation is from thirteen to seventeen years old. Often when we think about eating disorders, we think about anorexia nervosa, but this makes up only around 15% of all disorders. Others include bulimia, binge eating, food restriction, over-exercising and a preoccupation with food or an unhealthy obsession with a certain diet or approach to eating. Eating disorders do not just affect the individual but also cause severe distress for their loved ones. The priority is that these conditions are picked up as quickly as possible, with a prompt diagnosis, and responded to with early intervention, such as referral to a specialist as soon as an eating disorder is suspected, regardless of the girl's weight or body mass index (BMI).

Although eating disorders are a complex issue, it has been suggested that how adolescents *feel* about their body, rather than their actual weight, plays a more critical role in predicting whether they develop an eating disorder. We can all play an important role in positively influencing body-image pressures and managing expectations. The language we use about body size, bodyweight or aesthetics, and the value we attach to a certain bodyweight or appearance, can all have a big impact on an athlete's self-esteem and body image.

It's also important to consider that, as the converse of doing lots of training and not eating enough, there are also girls whose eating habits and lack of physical activity can cause too much weight gain, and this can also be a huge challenge. How do you support a teenage girl to lose weight or eat better without sending her into a downward spiral of dieting and extreme eating?

We must always start by acknowledging that, whether it's too much or too little food, as women we have a huge emotional relationship with food, which makes simply telling girls to eat more or eat less pretty futile. Establishing the reasons behind the eating behaviours, and talking these through with girls, or supporting them to talk this through with professionals, can be really helpful in making sense of what's going on and ultimately restoring healthy eating habits. Getting girls into the kitchen, preparing their own food and taking some of the responsibility for what they eat, can be empowering and educational, and can often help parents and girls reach compromises about what's on their plate.

We need to instil in girls from a really young age that it's not about being fat or thin, but about being healthy or unhealthy. Lean people can, because of their diets, be very unhealthy, and girls who carry slightly more weight, particularly as their body changes during puberty, can be very fit and healthy. It's hard to change this narrative, given how much girls are exposed to photoshopped images of lean, athletic bodies with no curves, no cellulite and washboard abs, or to thin supermodels. But things are changing; brands are realizing that it is their responsibility to depict healthy women of all shapes and sizes in their advertising, and the more visibility women's sport gets in the media, the more girls will have really positive role models who have strong, powerful bodies.

Encouraging girls to move

As well as lots of girls dropping out of sport completely by the end of their teens, another concern is that the majority of girls who do stay active in some way still don't meet recommended physical activity guidelines (according to a 2018 Sport England report).[7] And part of the problem happens way before bodies start changing in puberty. Researchers believe that most children – girls and boys – are developmentally capable of mastering all fundamental movement skills – things such as running, jumping, hopping, catching, throwing and kicking – by the time they are about ten years old.[8] They do this by being taught through appropriate activities, being given good demonstrations of skills, good feedback, and a variety of enjoyable and challenging practice activities. Yet despite the theory that boys and girls are capable of achieving mastery by the same age, girls consistently demonstrate poorer movement skills than boys, particularly in catching, throwing and kicking. In one study, only 14% of girls had mastered the kick and overarm throw on entering secondary school, compared with 50% of boys.[9]

When researchers try to explain the differences between boys and girls, they suggest that boys usually spend more time participating in different ball games and other activities that see them dashing about, falling over and physically larking around, compared with girls.[10] This makes a lot of sense, because although it's a bit of a cliché, in their spare time boys often are playing football with jumpers for goalposts or dodgeball with a tennis ball they found in a hedge. They play more invasion games, more games that require both locomotor skills – running, dodging, turning – and object-control skills – kicking, throwing, catching – than girls do. Research shows that in break times at school, girls prefer to engage in 'verbal' games rather than physical ones.[11] And there are more extra-curricular sports clubs available to boys than there are to girls, who tend to also spend more time in non-athletic pursuits after school, such as drama and music. All of this develops a movement-skill deficit. This is a barrier to participation in sport and exercise in the first place, and when women do get involved, it's another risk factor for injury. If we aren't developing movement skills in girls at a young age, how will they develop them at all?

Again, it's easy to point the finger at schools, since we know that school sport is under ever-increasing pressure, whether that's due to a lack of adequate facilities, staff numbers or PE being squeezed out of the timetable. But there are some great case studies of schools tackling the problem of girls not doing enough movement and physical activity in the Women's Sport and Fitness Foundation's 'Changing the Game, for Girls' teachers' toolkit.[12] Parents can play an important role here, too, by ensuring that the types of activities we encourage girls to get involved in, even at an early age, aren't being influenced by our unconscious gender biases. Let girls climb trees and get muddy, wrestle with siblings or play tag and 'stuck-in-the-mud', as opposed to ring-a-ring-a-roses and teddy bears' picnics, when we take them out to play. Research on parental expectations shows that parents unconsciously believe their sons are better than their daughters at sport, even when actual ability is the opposite. The consequence of this is that, over time, daughters absorb this belief and start to underestimate their own capabilities and potential. There are well-established links between self-belief, competence and the motivation to continue participating in sport. Parents, teachers and coaches all play vital roles in laying the foundation for a life-long relationship with physical activity in girls.

Let her find her spark

Helping girls find a sport or physical activity that they love is part of developing adolescents who are happy, positive and fearless. Research suggests that when interests and hobbies are supported by family, friends, school and community, teenagers develop more interpersonal communication and friend-making skills, more empathy and understanding of others' feelings, a better ability to work in teams and better psychological well-being and resilience.[13]

Supporting girls to find an active pursuit they love will help them thrive through puberty and in their life beyond. However, we have all seen the pushy parent in a sport or activity setting – the one who hasn't quite got the balance of encouragement and pressure right, where support spills over into frustration, where coaches and teachers get an earful, and girls are yelled at for not doing well enough. Steve Biddulph, psychologist and family therapist, reflects on how giving our kids enough space and time to find what they really love to do is a delicate balance. It doesn't mean crowding their spare time with lots of classes, sports and commitments, but being patient, perhaps even getting a little bored, while allowing their own inner confidence to emerge. Our job is to notice the interest, let them know we've seen it and that we're happy to support them in that pursuit.[14]

Research findings consistently show that teenage girls say that when sport stops being fun, they feel less inclined to stay involved. Extreme competitiveness and perfectionism can take the joy out of sport pretty quickly, even in girls who previously identified as sporty and were successful in their school or club environment. We want to keep the spark of love and enjoyment for training and performing alive in girls, while still being able to enjoy healthy competition and a desire for success. Perhaps there's a need to reinvigorate the idea that 'it's the taking part that matters' and reinforcing what girls can achieve beyond winning – enjoyment, personal development, building social connections, finding deep interests and passions for the game, as well as movement and using their bodies. Because when girls experience all these things, they are much more likely to fulfil their potential – not just their performance potential, but their potential to wholeheartedly live a happy and healthy life.

Education, education, education

Having conversations with girls, whether that's your daughter, niece, student or friend, raises their awareness and gives them important knowledge that can stand them in really good stead, not just during puberty, but when coping with what their body throws at them following childbirth or in perimenopause. A girl who is suffering from severe period pain in the first year of her cycles is going to cope much better knowing that there are things she can do about her symptoms, that her symptoms might change as she gets older, and that this isn't necessarily her lot for the rest of her life. Educating girls around good breast support means that breast pain related to her cycle, or embarrassment about breasts moving, are removed as reasons that girls might opt out of being active, both now and in the future. Knowing how hormones can influence our brain as well as our body can help girls navigate changing moods and motivations in puberty, but also during the hormonal roller coaster of perimenopause. Simply put, when young women learn more about their body during puberty, they become better ambassadors for their health and well-being across the rest of their life.

How to be well in puberty

- Puberty is a very 'vulnerable' life stage but we can help girls celebrate the amazing things that are happening within their bodies.
- Be a stable presence that girls can come back to as their hormones roller-coaster along, their bodies change and their emotions become confusing.
- Be positive: check your own biases and attitudes to your body before you impart them on others.
- Get girls moving more, earlier. Let them move through play and expose them to all the activities boys do. They must learn to move their bodies well.

- Educate girls about nutrition and support good attitudes towards it, based on feeling healthy and having energy, rather than looking skinny.
- Don't encourage girls to specialize in one sport too early, as it can lead to over-use injuries, burnout and drop-out.
- Be patient if girls are still finding out how they love to move. Don't catastrophize changes in bodies or skill levels during puberty; this is a transitory phase and putting someone in a box in terms of ability, sportiness or performance is impotent during such a time of change. Let her enjoy her sport, her body. The rest will follow.

Moving through midlife

Midlife, generally accepted as being between the ages of forty-five and fifty-five, is the most common time for a woman to begin the transition into perimenopause, when periods become irregular, menstrual cycle hormones can fluctuate wildly and start declining overall as women approach menopause. A woman is considered to have reached the menopause once periods have stopped for a full year. A good way to look at these stages is that it's the opposite of puberty. If puberty is when your hormones are getting themselves ready to have a regular cycle, perimenopause is the time when they are winding down and your body is getting ready to stop having your cycle.

Five years ago, the word menopause was barely a whisper in the media or online; in fact, this inevitable life stage for women was often surrounded by shame and embarrassment. A 2022 Fawcett Society report uncovered the stigma many women face, with 41% saying that they have seen menopause or menopause symptoms treated as a joke by people at work.[15] There has been a gap in research, in awareness and in medical training for menopause care, and many women and their families suffer in silence, not knowing what to expect or how to access help.

But things are changing. Research and up-to-date, evidence-based training is improving, we are hearing more about the menopause in the media and online, and it is now on the curriculum to be taught in schools. A recent survey by Joyce Harper, a professor of reproductive science at the Institute for Women's Health, University College London, showed that 90% of women had never been taught about the menopause at school, 60% of women didn't feel informed at all about it and 30% of women were 'dreading' it.[16]

But it's not all doom and gloom. Early education and awareness of the menopause is key so that women can be in control, as opposed to waiting for the menopause to take charge of them, and Professor Harper is trying to encourage women to see menopause in a different, more positive light. Postmenopause is a time when women don't have to manage periods or menstrual cycle symptoms. For those women who have suffered with hormone-sensitive symptoms for their fertile lives, such as endometriosis or polycystic ovarian syndrome, they might now be symptom-free. There are many medication options available for women during the menopause, such as hormone replacement therapy (HRT), but lifestyle and exercise is, as always, fundamental in keeping well and happy in this life stage.

A hormonal roller coaster

During perimenopause, you've gone from having a lovely, natural cycle that's kind of predictable and inevitable in terms of what the hormones do across the month, to being slightly more chaotic, with an overall decline in both oestrogen and progesterone. Just as the rising hormone levels affect us physically and emotionally during the menstrual cycle, rapidly declining hormones also have an impact, often with more erratic highs and lows – and lower lows than ever. All of this contributes to how we feel and the symptoms we experience. Perimenopausal symptoms can last for up to ten years, although the average length is about four years.[17]

While erratic but declining oestrogen and progesterone are the defining features of our hormonal midlife, other important hormones are slowing down, too, which can compound symptoms and affect our get-up-and-go when it comes to exercise. Women produce testosterone in lower levels than men, but it's still an important hormone in women's bodies and it, too, declines as we age. This drop-off in testosterone can cause symptoms of low libido, profound tiredness, lack of motivation and muscle weakness, and researchers have found that testosterone replacement (the experiments were conducted in women who'd had surgically-induced menopause) improves muscle mass and muscle strength, which in turn improve physical function in women.[18]

Melatonin, a hormone that controls our sleep–wake cycle and influences mood and immune function, also noticeably declines during midlife. Insomnia is a commonly reported symptom during perimenopause, and while it can occur due to other symptoms, such as night sweats, anxiety and restlessness, getting in the way of sleep, declining levels of hormones such as melatonin are also thought to directly impact sleep.[19] This has led researchers to investigate whether taking melatonin supplements can improve sleep in menopausal women, but the conclusion is currently that topping up melatonin doesn't improve sleep or mood in midlife women.[20] This really reflects how complex the whole hormonal system is during menopause, and that just adding in one hormone isn't enough. It's about finding what combination of diet, exercise, supplementation and, possibly, HRT medication works for you.

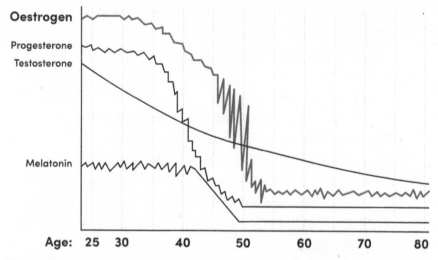

Oestrogen
Progesterone
Testosterone

Melatonin

Age: 25 30 40 50 60 70 80

Fluctuating hormones across our life stages. The graph shows the erratic and declining hormones as we enter midlife and go through the perimenopause in our forties and early fifties, and the low levels of hormones after menopause.

Menopause 101

- Menopause is an inevitable stage in every woman's life, when her periods stop, and it happens to most women in their late forties or early fifties.
- The menopause can begin in one of three ways:
    a) Naturally, when the ovaries gradually shut down and stop ovulating.
    b) Medically, when medication switches off the ovaries.
    c) Surgically, when the ovaries are surgically removed.
- A natural menopause is preceded by the perimenopause, which is often referred to as the 'hormonal roller coaster'. It's when you get the majority of symptoms, which can last from two to ten years.

- There can be some confusion between the different terms for the menopause. The 'menopause' tends to be the umbrella term for this overall life stage, but more specifically:
  a) The perimenopause is the time when you have menopause symptoms but you're still having periods, whether regular or irregular.
  b) The menopause is when your periods have stopped for one year (if you're over fifty) or two (if you're over forty-five).
  c) The postmenopause is the time after the menopause.
- Midlife is a stressful time of life for everyone, regardless of your life circumstances, and lifestyle choices can have a hugely positive impact on your ability to cope.
- Every woman's experience of her perimenopause and menopause will be different. Symptoms can differ vastly, as can their severity and the impact they have on the lives of the woman and her family.
- 80% of women will experience hot flushes, with insomnia, weight gain and brain fog other prevalent symptoms – but there are literally hundreds of reported symptoms.
- Guidelines from the National Institute for Health and Care Excellence (NICE) recommend hormone replacement therapy (HRT) for nearly all women, and your doctor will be able to prescribe this. More and more women are benefiting from HRT, which can have short- and long-term benefits. In the short term, supplementary oestrogen can help with the symptoms of the menopause and in the long term it can help protect our bones, hearts, bowels, skin, mind and so much more. There is a small increased risk of breast cancer with taking HRT, and so it's important

to discuss this with the healthcare professional who is prescribing it.

- Currently HRT prescribed in the UK is body-identical, which means it's almost identical to the hormone naturally produced in a woman's body, so it's very well tolerated.
- Not everyone can take, needs to take or wants to take HRT, and there are non-hormonal medications that can be prescribed by your doctor.
- It's important not to forget testosterone. Low testosterone can cause symptoms of low libido and profound tiredness, and women who experience these can benefit from taking testosterone replacement.
- Exercise (both aerobic and strength work) has been described as the only non-controversial beneficial aspect of lifestyle modification during menopause, and it should feature in all women's lives.
- The British Menopause Society website is a great resource of evidence-based advice and also has a list of recognized menopause specialists, both private and NHS. Another great resource is the Balance app, created by Dr Louise Newson, a doctor, menopause specialist and menopause campaigner.
- There are supplements you can try to relieve menopause symptoms, including magnesium, vitamin D and agnus castus. There is little evidence supporting other supplements, such as black cohosh, red clover and sage, among other herbal remedies, but our ethos is this: if you find that it helps you, that it doesn't do you harm and that it doesn't cost the earth, then go for it.

Bella

I see many women on a daily basis with menopause symptoms, and more and more who are keen to take HRT. A fifty-three-year-old woman who worked long hours with a daily commute had, until relatively recently, managed her stressful life with running and regular exercise. One day she came to see me in tears because she was concerned she had dementia. She described being in meetings where she would suddenly lose her train of thought, her mind would go blank and she was unable to finish her sentence. This made her panicky and worsened her anxiety. After further questioning, it turned out she was having other symptoms, too, including hot flushes and night sweats, and had become unable to exercise for months due to fatigue. She'd wake up feeling exhausted and was unable to do her usual self-care routine; the wheels had come off her lifestyle. She was unable to find the time or the energy to make home-cooked meals and was drinking too much wine in the evenings. This would have a knock-on effect the next day and things were spiralling out of control.

The woman was shocked to learn that her symptoms were likely due to the perimenopause, and she was understandably relieved to learn that it was not dementia. She started some oestrogen gel HRT that you apply to your skin and leave to absorb (don't rub it in – let it sink in naturally!), and for progesterone, she chose to have a hormonal coil inserted. Within a few weeks of using the HRT gel, she started to feel better, and the first thing she noticed was the improved sleep. She finally felt able to get her lifestyle back on track, back to running regularly and drinking less alcohol.

Thankfully, awareness of the menopause has come on leaps and bounds over the past few years, with books and documentaries openly discussing the symptoms and range of remedies available, so many more women know what to look out for and when to seek help.

Midlife superwoman

Women in midlife really want to be active but face a unique set of barriers that differ in the context of every woman's body, and her life. Whether it's the midlife physiology that you have to overcome, or the logistics and responsibilities that come with being a forty- or fifty-something-year-old woman, we know that at this stage of life finding a balance can feel hard. Finding time for yourself can feel hard. Fitting in the exercise that everyone tells you will make you feel better feels hard. While midlife brings some pretty amazing features for women, a lot of it is pretty darn hard.

Some midlife women have always loved sport and training – they grew up watching *Gladiators* on a Saturday evening, had sporting role models such as Sally Gunnell, Steffi Graf and Sharron Davies, and grew up at a time when girls and women could do a lot of sport and exercise. This generation is now hitting midlife and still loves to work out hard and even compete. But they do so in a system that doesn't have the knowledge or programmes in place to best support them. Their bodies are changing, and what used to work for them in terms of getting them fit, keeping them fit and maintaining a healthy body composition, is no longer doing the job. For women who have been tuned in to their bodies and how to get the best out of them for decades, this can be a really upsetting and frustrating reality.

Other midlife women might have given up on sport in their

youth, labelling themselves as 'not sporty', or they didn't return to exercise after having children. For women in this group who want to start or get back to exercise, to combat the menopausal weight gain, the physical or emotional symptoms of changing hormones, or to manage the stress of life, there is very little information or support available, and the whole process can feel intimidating. It's often easier to keep avoiding the idea completely. When women do restart sport – say, by giving net-ball another go or joining a gym – they often don't enjoy it because it doesn't feel good – it feels precarious, their body doesn't feel designed for physical activity, they feel they might get injured quickly or they don't feel at home among a group of younger women. But when these women find an activity they enjoy, when they find a group or a setting where they feel welcome and supported, and not judged or criticized, it's amazing to watch the physical improvements and the vitality that it brings.

Exercise classes, personal trainers, coaches and even online workouts rarely focus on helping midlife women get the best out of their bodies, push their fitness or combat the symptoms of age or the menopause. Midlife women either have to fit in to programmes that have been designed for bodies that are not theirs, or they are relegated to the lighter, more amiable workouts such as yoga and aqua aerobics (absolutely nothing wrong with these, by the way; they're just not the only exercise that we should be encouraging midlife women to do).

Baz has trained hundreds of midlife women and has found there are some key areas to focus on. At The Well HQ, our fundamental belief is that women need to move and, importantly, to find movement that they enjoy (you don't have to love it, but you do have to enjoy it or it won't stick). During midlife, exercise is arguably as important, if not more so, than any time of life, because not only can exercise help to manage many of the symptoms associated with the perimenopause, it also has longer-term effects on our cardiac, bone, muscle and psychological health that no drugs can offer. Our mobility, independence and happiness in old age relies pretty heavily on the attitude we take to moving our bodies during our midlife.

Whether you're looking to record a lifetime 10km PB or you're embarking on a Couch to 5K programme, there are things you can do as an active midlife woman that will help you get the best out of your body.

- **Track your symptoms**
  Track everything! From your menstrual cycle, sleep, hot flushes, aches, pains and energy levels to how exercise feels and your changing appetite. The more information you have, the more impactful any proposed solutions will be. It also means you are far more attuned to your body and have body literacy, which is such a good tool when it comes to navigating the menopause.

- **Master managing your periods**
  Periods during perimenopause can be really heavy (thanks to abnormally high oestrogen levels during your cycle) or arrive unexpectedly (cycles tend to shorten in early perimenopause, but cycles can also be longer one month then shorter the next). Period underwear can be useful if you aren't really sure when your bleed will arrive (you can wear it 'just in case') and can also be used as back-up for tampons if you're experiencing very heavy bleeds. Menstrual cups can be a great way to manage heavy periods, too, as they can collect more blood than a single tampon and are safe to leave in for up to twelve hours.

- **Talk about your pelvic floor with someone who can help**
  On average, it takes women seven years to ask for help with their stress incontinence, yet it's a classic midlife

conversation among friends; pelvic floor symptoms, including leaking or bladder and bowel issues, typically start or get worse at this time.

- **Know the elephant in your room**
Our bodies may become more sensitive to alcohol, sugar and caffeine as we enter midlife. If these are features of your diet, it could be triggering some of your symptoms. Try taking these out of your diet and seeing what happens. If these are the elephant in your room, you need to deal with it. No amount of kale, activated almonds or salmon is going to counteract your gin and tonic habit – it's just not!

- **Look at your training objectively**
Your existing training programmes may not work so well for you any more. Long endurance sessions can be more exhausting than they once were, and faster interval sessions may feel better. These shorter, sharper sessions are a key consideration for midlife women because they tick a lot of boxes in terms of bone health and muscle strength, provided your pelvic floor can tolerate the impact. Be aware of the impact different sessions have on your sleep and anxiety levels too, and how much recovery you need to feel ready to train again. Become attuned to what works for your whole self.

- **Warm up**
Because we're more prone to injury during perimenopause, it's really important to do a progressive warm-up for at least ten minutes before you start any runs, HIIT sessions or any other vigorous activity. Not only does it prepare your muscles for what's to come, it also tells your nervous system that you're getting ready to go, rather than shocking your system and kick-starting a stress response.

- **Lift weights**

  Strength work is good for bones, body shape and muscles. As we get older, our muscle mass decreases by 3–8% per decade over the age of thirty.[21] By working with weights or adding carefully constructed HIIT sessions that feature bodyweight-resistance exercises, you can help to maintain or increase your muscle mass and you can alter your body mass composition so that you reduce fat percentage in favour of muscle. This is not only great for your metabolism, and offsetting potential weight gain, but women with more muscle mass have been shown to have a reduction in menopause symptoms such as hot flushes.[22]

  Strength training also helps prevent injuries by strengthening and balancing muscles, and by keeping bones strong. Another tick in the box for strength training during this phase of life is that research has shown that women who lift heavy weights are at reduced risk of prolapse.[23] However, you must learn to strength-train well, with good technique that allows you to maximize the gains and not exacerbate any potential issues. You can find a guide to strength exercises in Chapter 7 – see 'Bodies that move well'. If you have access to a trainer in your gym, book in a session to learn proper weightlifting techniques. There's nothing better for your confidence to lift than being coached how to do these strength exercises correctly at the start. The majority of strength and conditioning programmes can be adapted for back pain (very common in women by this age) and to minimize the risk of pelvic floor dysfunction, which can be brought on by the increase in abdominal pressure caused by holding your breath. Work with a trainer who knows what they're doing and find one who can support your individual needs. It's not just physically that you will reap the benefits of strength training; research shows that when performed regularly, strength work reduces anxiety and stress, and improves symptoms of depression.[24]

- **Really recover**
  As we age, we need more recovery time from exercise, and recovery becomes more vital for restoring our energy levels, repairing our muscles and resetting us for the next workout. Exercise in midlife is about training smarter, not harder. This can be tough to get your head around if you have always exercised in a particular way – doing less to get more can seem counterintuitive. Midlife is a great time to give yourself permission to do that, so you can benefit from the training and exercise that you're doing. Ways to do this are to have more recovery days in the week, do fewer morning sessions and also to include whole recovery weeks more often (every two to three weeks). You'll know if you have your recovery right as you'll be getting the results you'd expect, have loads of energy for your 'exercise' sessions and not have to drag yourself through them.

- **Fuelling your exercise matters in midlife, too**
  Midlife women have different nutritional needs when it comes to energy and exercise. They can't metabolize fructose (fruit sugar) and turn it into energy very well, so avoid sports drinks and other carb-heavy sports nutrition. There's also a greater sensitivity to carbs, which can mean more blood-sugar peaks and troughs, causing chaos for mood and appetite. Stick to wholegrains and veggies for your carbs and increase your protein. You need more protein because your body is now using it less effectively.

- **Harness your hydration**
  When it comes to staying energized throughout your workout, hydration is key. We don't handle heat as well

during the menopause, so hydration is also a key strategy to help the body stay cool. Even if you're worried about your pelvic floor, make sure you still drink. Drinking less does not mean you'll leak less!

- **Ask for help early**
Women wait too long to seek out help. We don't prioritize seeing someone about our symptoms, or we minimize them and convince ourselves everything's fine; that we would be wasting a doctor's time. If you're in your forties and your cycle has shortened or you're experiencing other symptoms, the first call for support should be to your doctor to discuss general advice and explore options such as HRT or lifestyle changes. You should also consider finding a women's health practitioner for pelvic floor checks. It's unnecessary to have costly testing or expensive HRT treatments. If you want to go private then, if possible, get assessed independently as opposed to at a clinic with a range of products or services that they'll want to sell you.

Baz

I recently worked with a woman in her late forties who enjoyed running and training for marathons. She got up early every day and ran before work. She came to me because she was getting irresistible urges to urinate while out on her runs, and it was ruining her enjoyment of running. Apart from this, she was managing pretty well with the menopause and its symptoms. We removed potential bladder irritants in her diet and worked on her pelvic floor dynamics, and things started to improve for her. But after four weeks, she went for a run and experienced the same kind of urges as before. I was a bit flummoxed because I couldn't work out the cause of this – until I asked about vaginal oestrogen, which she said she'd just stopped using the previous weekend as she wasn't sure she needed it any more. That was the ta-da moment. The vaginal oestrogen – which is a very small, targeted dose of oestrogen applied directly to the vagina – had been plumping up her vagina enough for it to support her bladder, so she wasn't getting the urges to urinate while running. Without the vaginal oestrogen, her symptoms came back.

Because this isn't a substantial medical issue, this woman might have just decided her body was no longer built for running. But menopause symptoms, however insignificant they seem for one person, can be life-altering for another. For my client it was huge, and because we had a relationship where she was happy to talk about anything and everything, we got her back on the vaginal oestrogen and she returned to enjoying her running without worrying about the location of the closest toilet. A woman's exercise routine can be slowed or even stopped because of life-changing symptoms. Don't let these changes stop you moving or showing up to clubs or classes that you've been enjoying for years. With a little bit of knowledge, some attention to your symptoms and suitable remedies, you can continue doing what you love and reap the benefits for much longer.

What if you want a natural midlife with no drugs?

Women often say they would rather 'go through the menopause naturally' or try to do it 'without medication'. It's fantastic when an individual optimizes their lifestyle and diet, especially if this alone resolves all their symptoms. It is important, however, that women who still have symptoms continue to seek help from their doctor or a menopause specialist.

If we women could only think about the menopause differently and consider it as 'oestrogen deficiency', we might be more empathetic to each other and receptive to support. If you're experiencing moderate to severe symptoms, despite lifestyle adjustments, then it's likely that your body is low on oestrogen and you may benefit from hormone replacement. That's OK. In fact, it's great that there is an easily accessible, safe remedy available to you. When diabetics find out their insulin – another hormone – is deficient, most don't hesitate when offered medication to help restore the effects of insulin, manage their symptoms and allow them to live a full life. It's not that the menopause is a disease, or that every woman should be medicated through her midlife. But there is medication to help you get your body in balance and you don't need to suffer with your symptoms on a daily basis. At The Well HQ, we have seen so many women reject the idea of HRT because they see using it as a weakness, or have concerns over its safety, and this stops them getting the help they need and that they would benefit from greatly.

FAQs

Every woman's health-and-fitness regime is different, and the menopause affects each woman's relationship with exercise in different ways. Here are some of the questions we commonly get asked about moving our bodies in midlife and our answers to get your body moving.

My back keeps flaring up. I don't like going to the gym but love sport, and I just feel like my body is letting me down like it's never done before. I don't trust it.

Back pain and joint pain in general is very common. Get curious about this niggle so you can understand what makes it better or worse. At this stage of life, it won't just magically get better. Movement and exercise is good, but not when you're in pain, and although you know this, some specific rehabilitation work either with a physio, personal trainer or Pilates is probably going to be worth it. If you can't justify the cost or time, just think of what you would say to a friend or family member who was in your position – and follow your own advice!

I've put on weight and no matter how hard I train, it's not shifting.

You may need to do less exercise. Midlife is stressful and stress is an inflammatory state for our bodies to be in, meaning that you're less likely to lose weight if you're stressed. Take a step back, and make sure you're not always training early morning without breakfast or making all of your sessions really hard. Build in exercise sessions that involve stretching, walking in nature, wild swimming, yoga – all of this will 'down train' your systems and help get you out of that fight-and-flight mode.

I'm a marathon runner, but I'm exhausted from all the training. I want to get a PB and know I can, but I'm not sure how.

You may need to run less, vary your training, eat better and sleep more. We suggest building in a good-quality strength and conditioning programme. Shifting from six good runs a week to four brilliant ones, with two to three targeted strength sessions, can help you to build strength, reduce your injury risk and improve your running form. It's a big shift in mentality but it's an approach that's proven to work.

I love wild swimming. What else should I be doing?

Keep doing what you love but have a think about ways of doing some circuit-type training. Try doing this before your swim; you don't have to go to a special venue but including some strength training two to three times a week would be excellent.

I want to start doing weights. Where should I start?

If you've never lifted anything before, start with your own body-weight through exercises like squats and push-ups, and focus very intentionally on technique. Wire your brain so that it knows the right movement patterns to do in squats and lunges, so when you do eventually add weight and try more advanced moves, your movement patterns will be right and you'll reduce your risk of injury. Don't skip forward too soon, but when you're feeling confident with your technique, move up to some light dumb-bells and resistance bands before moving to bigger weights. If you want to go to a gym, then machine weights could also be a great place to build up your confidence to get started. Even three times a week is fantastic. Your priority should be to get some input from someone who knows what they're doing to teach you safe lifting techniques.

I'm thinking of doing my first triathlon. Is it sensible to start such a strenuous new sporting hobby in midlife?

Go for it! Pick a sprint triathlon for starters and register – that way, you've paid your money and you're more likely to get your-self organized and start training for it. Local clubs are usually great at helping you prepare for your first triathlon. To start with, focus on making a plan for your training. Sports like triath-lon are notorious for lack of recovery, just because you have to fit three sports into your training. So, when you plan your schedule, make sure you feature rest in that plan, plus a couple of strength-training sessions a week. Training in a group of friends, or at a club, will help with motivation and enjoyment.

I used to be brilliant at sport, but I'm not sure I can cope with starting again and I'm feeling disappointed by not being as good as I used to be.

You need to be kind to yourself. It's easier said than done, but honestly, it's a case of saying, 'OK, this is who I am right now, this is how much I'm doing in my life and I'm not going to beat myself up about how many burpees I do (or don't do).' Go and do what you want to do, focus on you, start moving, and you'll love it.

How to be well in menopause

- Your body is changing. How you approached diet and exercise in your twenties and thirties might not serve you as well in your forties or fifties. Be prepared to relearn what works best for you.
- This is a stressful time, regardless of your life circumstances. If you do one thing, work on managing that stress. Exercise can be super-helpful here, but done wrong, it can add to the bad biology that stress creates.
- Lifestyle really helps – you'll likely need to review and rewrite how you do things, but once you build new habits, you will feel the benefits, physically and emotionally.
- Build strength. It's the most overlooked aspect of being fit, resilient and happy from midlife onwards. It's a game changer.
- Ask for help early – the sooner the better. Use NHS menopause doctors and clinics and, if your resources allow

it, you can explore private clinics and complementary health therapies.

- It's potentially the only life stage that you can be really well prepared for – there is plenty of information out there, so arm yourself with knowledge and a toolbox of strategies. Like any life stage, we don't know what our experience will be in the end, but the more prepared and empowered we are, the better we can advocate for our own health and well-being.

- Midlife doesn't mean getting ready for the end of your life. For many, it's a time of new-found freedom. If you had children, they may have flown the nest; you may have more time to spend doing what you love; you develop a new resilience, and a much lower bar for tolerating BS. You can fall in love with your body without the insecurities of youth. You are your own person.

Chapter 12

Where We Belong

In this book we've given you what we believe is fundamentally yours: knowledge about your brilliant body and how what's going on with it can influence how you experience the world and pursue your goals. But knowing more about your body doesn't automatically make you a better architect of your own health and wellness. Knowing more and not taking action won't result in positive change. You have to develop habits that support health and wellness, and we hope that the knowledge you've gained by reading this book helps you do so.

Unfortunately, it's not your journey to take alone. You don't exist in a vacuum. We all occupy a space in the centre of an overlapping Venn diagram of ecosystems – an ecosystem of family and friends; of peers, colleagues and work; one of our online world; one of society now, and one of the society that came before. It doesn't matter if we're talking about unleashing the power of food or our hormones, being more open about periods or pelvic floors, or finding the perfect bra – being able to do any of these things is influenced by the beliefs and actions of everyone and everything within those ecosystems. They mould and shape us, often without our permission. And when we come up short, when we feel our body is letting us down or think that we're just not cut out for doing something, please remember that it's probably not you, not your body, not your ability to endure the human condition. It's those ecosystems that have failed you: the deeply held beliefs about women; the structural silencing of women's pain; the lack of education about our bodies through our lives; the division of resources away from researching women's health and their experiences; the inequality of women in sport. In short, the patriarchy.

The fabric of our world

The physical environment that surrounds us affects how we go about our lives and how smooth our experience of being a woman is on any given day. Take toilets. When a man goes to the toilet, he needs a vessel to go in (usually a urinal or a toilet), and if he's done a poo, he'll need some toilet roll. But for a woman, a vessel and some toilet roll is rarely enough. At any one time, 800 million girls and women worldwide are on their period, and what a woman needs at this time is a vessel to go in, toilet roll (not just for poo), period products, and somewhere safe and hygienic to dispose of her used period products or a place to empty and wash out her menstrual cup. Although many women carry spare supplies with them, in a survey of American women 86% said they started their period unexpectedly at work without the products they needed, and of those, over 60% left work to buy products and 34% went home to get what they needed.[1] Having your period can therefore not only be embarrassing, frustrating and a hassle; it's damaging productivity and performance, because time is lost from the working day to sort it out.

Sports clubs and exercise facilities are often the worst culprits. Sometimes there are simply no toilets at all, whether that's at an outside setting for a circuit class or at a race or competition venue. In all our experience, from fun runs to marathons, at an open water swim or charity bike ride, while men are peeing in bushes, women are queuing up for ages outside the two portable toilets that have been cordially provided for hundreds of women participating that day. And if portable toilets are involved, then they often lack a way to dispose of period products. We've heard from women who have turned up to play at their weekly league match to find only one toilet for thirty women to share (you guessed it – the other toilet facilities were a row of urinals). Or we're at places where sanitary bins are full and overflowing with used products, or they're broken, so you can't lift the lid hygienically with the pedal.

For everyone to have an equal experience of using the toilet, everyone should be confident that when they use the facilities available, they'll have everything they need. It sounds simple, doesn't it? Yet, even if a venue manages to have a clean toilet, with loo paper and a working period-product bin, few places have period products available in the toilet, the washroom facilities or the changing rooms.

There are many reasons a woman might get caught short coming on her period without having the products she needs – and laziness or disorganization are rarely among them, as has been suggested to us by people who don't want to put 'freebies' in the toilets because, well, it costs money. The menstrual cycle can be affected by a range of factors, including age, diet, training, travel, stress, and the fact that periods can just be less regular in some women, varying by up to eight days each month. Offering period products in toilet facilities lifts this stress from a woman's life. It also keeps her from leaving wherever she has found herself caught short. If you turn up to an exercise class and find you've come on, but you aren't confident to ask around and there are no period products available, it's likely you'll have to leave to get hold of something and risk missing your class or your opportunity to be active for that day. Not having period products freely available at best causes added angst, and at worst is a barrier to exercise. The truth is that it's not that expensive for the facilities' management to provide products. Aside from the fact that in

1984 NASA famously sent a hundred tampons into space for Sally Ride's seven-day space flight (just to be safe), women typically take only what they need in that moment, which will be one product, at the most two. The cost of this would be about £3.50 per woman annually and is unlikely to exceed the huge gain in well-being for the girls and women in their moment of need.[2]

Scotland is ahead of the rest of the UK on this.[3] In November 2020 Scotland became the first country in the world to provide free and universal access to period products. The Period Products (Free Provision) (Scotland) Act was passed unanimously through the Scottish Parliament, requiring period products be made available for all those who need them, including at schools, sports clubs, entertainment venues, and restaurants. Even before this legislation was passed, sportscotland offered a small grant to sports clubs to make products available to their female members free of charge.

There are some places, like the great outdoors, where managing periods becomes trickier because there's no toilet. Whether you're rambling, geo-caching, hiking, cycling or exploring, having a period and nowhere to manage it can be a barrier to enjoying these pursuits for women. Adventurer and endurance athlete Anna McNuff told us, 'It's something that actually stops many women taking to the outdoors, or feeling comfortable when they do. In the twenty-first century, that's rather ridiculous. We need more innovation, more talk, so more women are comfortable and happy on adventures.' Fortunately, innovation is happening. Menstrual cups and period underwear reduce the need for disposable period products that need changing frequently, so you can be out and about all day and not have to find a place to change and dispose of products. For women who use tampons or pads, the invention of biodegradable yet hard-working period-product disposal bags enables you to carry your used period product safely sealed in your pocket or bag, without fear of mess or odour, and to dispose of it later on.[4] We spoke to a teacher who said inventions such as these have been brilliant for girls doing their Duke of Edinburgh expeditions, who had previously been terrified of what to do if they were on their period for their trek.

Beyond facilities, women have also been getting a raw deal when it comes to sport and exercise kit and equipment. In 2019, Hannah Dines openly discussed the vulval injury she sustained from years of elite cycling, having spent so many hours training on a saddle designed for a man, which put pressure on her vulva as she adopted a racing position on her bike. Our vulva isn't meant to be a weight-bearing part of our anatomy, and over time, Hannah experienced pain and swelling. In the end, scar tissue started to develop that needed to be surgically removed. It's crazy that even at the elite level, women don't have equipment that's been designed for a female body, and even more so that Hannah's initial complaints about the pain were dismissed as normal saddle-soreness. This is why it's so important to know what's normal and what's not, and to feel comfortable using the names for the part of your anatomy that's hurting. It's a very different thing having pain or an abrasion on your buttocks or perineum (the bit between your anus and genitalia) than it is to have pain and swelling in your vulva. Being able to articulate the problem helps get to a solution more quickly. Bike kit designers have slowly recognized the need for female-specific saddles, and a range of brands have now designed some. The ideal women's saddle is broader on the seat to support wider seat bones in women, with a large cut-out, or relief channel, running down the middle, so there's no pressure put on the vulva when the rider adopts a forward position. Because every woman is different, it will still take a checklist of your body shape, your riding position preference, riding style and your bike fit to find a perfect match for you, but knowing that you need a saddle designed for a woman's body is a great start.

And if elite cyclists struggle to get a good saddle fit, it's unsurprising that Miss Jo Average is at even greater risk of riding on a saddle that isn't designed for her and has the potential to cause harm. Take indoor cycling bikes, with smart-fitness technology and screens for online classes as an example. These have grown in popularity and are used as much by women as by men. They often come with a range of specially designed accessories, including shoes, heart rate monitors, weights and a water bottle. But at the time of writing, none come with an option for a women's saddle. It doesn't make sense that this kind of thing is overlooked, but time and time again, it is. With the convenience of this type of workout – home-based and time-flexible – there is even greater risk that women will be spending a significant amount of time on their indoor bikes getting super-fit and healthy, but with a broken vulva. A friend of ours found her own solution and bought an inexpensive gel saddle cover, which helped alleviate some of the pain she experienced. An inexpensive cover on an expensive bike, just to make it work for her. Big brands need to commit to diligently exploring whether the equipment and kit they design and sell with the promise of health and fitness really works for women's bodies. And if it doesn't, make an equally priced, equally available solution that does.

It's not just technical equipment like bike saddles that may be poorly designed for women. Even things like gym benches have been designed with men in mind – they're too long and often too high for women, so instead of a woman being able to lie correctly on her back for a chest-press exercise, allowing her feet to touch the floor, she will often be forced to adopt an arched back position when lifting – an incorrect technique that puts her at greater risk of injury. Weight-lifting women: the quick fix here is to make sure you put your feet on a yoga block, some weight plates or an aerobics step, so that you can comfortably plant your feet while keeping good form on the bench. The same rule applies to all gym equipment – it's likely been designed to accommodate a man's grip, frame and physique. If you find that a certain machine or exercise is causing you to lose form, it may be the design of the equipment and you may have to seek help in finding an alternative exercise or to use a strategy to adjust your position on the equipment.

Lydia Greenway, former England cricketer, was fed up with the lack of equipment and kit designed for girls and women in her sport. In an interview with the *Cricketer*, Lydia recalled, 'Our England shirts used to be so big it was as if we were wearing parachutes. Fortunately, over the years that has changed because they recognized that the female body shape is different.'[5] Lydia is determined to make kit and equipment offerings inclusive in a sport that has traditionally only provided kit designed for males, so when girls wanted to play they had to get a 'small boys' size. To that end, she works with brands to design female-specific kit for softball and hardball cricket and sells these online.[6]

Cricket is certainly not the only sport to have waited a long time for kit designed specifically for women. The 2019 FIFA Women's World Cup was the first time the women wore kit specifically designed for them, rather than wearing derivatives of the men's kit, and also the first time that a sports bra was included in the kit bag from sponsor Nike. But for those not playing at the World Cup, the club offerings are still leaving women feeling like the younger sister wearing the older brother's hand-me-downs. Karin Legemate, a retired Dutch professional football player, found that at a first-division club, the sponsor didn't have a line of women's clothing, so she had to play in the smallest men's size and, because the smallest size of the men's boots was bigger than her shoe size, in children's shoes.[7] Because competitions are waged mentally as well as physically, in sport, Karin experienced her oversized, ill-fitting men's kit as a huge impediment – it looked wrong; it felt wrong. The children's boots had plastic, rather than aluminium, studs, so with their reduced grip she couldn't turn as well. Her standard of play was impacted. It's like starting a match one–nil down before the first whistle even blows, because your kit hasn't been designed for your body.

In one of the most high-profile women's rugby-club league games of its time, called 'The Big Game' in 2021, Harlequins women's team appeared to be wearing match-day shirts that were too big. The club later responded to questions about the kit by Fi Tomas of the *Telegraph* by saying the shirts were made by Adidas in 'one fit, for both men's and women's teams'. The reality is that 'one fit' means 'men's fit'. How are women meant to feel like they belong in sport when they are made to wear kit that's designed for a man's body? For professional sports clubs, the argument is often that the brand supplying all the kit doesn't make a woman's version, so the men and women have to wear the same fit – the men's. We've spoken to many football and rugby players who have challenged that school of thought, saying that if it's OK for men and women to wear the same fit, why don't we buy all the kit as women's fit, and the men can play in that? As you can imagine, that idea goes down like a lead balloon – but why should it? It's exactly the same situation, except this time it's the men who are playing in kit that's not optimized for their bodies. But apparently that's out of the question.

It's not just at the top levels of women's rugby that these problems arise. In a survey of women playing the sport in England by the Girls Rugby Club in 2020, some 83% of women said they had experienced issues with the size and fit of their supplied rugby kit, and 69% felt girls and women were not adequately catered for when it came to buying rugby playing and training kit. There are often cost implications for grassroots clubs providing different kit for the boys' and girls' teams. If that's your club, then why not get a crowdfunding project set up or organize a fundraising event so that the girls in the club can feel like they belong in their sport, rather than living in the oversized shirt-shadow of the boys' teams? And if your beloved sport doesn't have at least some offering of kit and equipment designed for women, tell them about it! The omission is not usually a conspiracy; it's an upsetting oversight borne out of sport being designed *by* men *for* men. With few women in leadership roles around boardroom tables in the sporting world, it's not surprising that facilities and equipment sometimes lack female insight. Social media gives us an amazing platform to connect with brands to tell them what we love, and to tell them when they could do better. If they need to do better at providing for women in their sports, tell them!

Kit designed for men is one thing, but even when kit *is* made 'for women', it doesn't truly seem to be made with women's bodies in mind. One football club we worked with wondered for a long time why the players loved their away kit so much, even though it wasn't as fancy as the home kit. The reason was because the shorts weren't white; they were navy blue. And girls who were worried about leaking when on their period, or starting their period unexpectedly, hated having to wear white shorts and felt a massive load of unnecessary stress was taken off when they could wear darker-coloured shorts for away matches. White and light-coloured kit, or kits that are too tight and clingy, are reasons that girls don't do sport. In a survey by hockey player and researcher Tess Howard, 75% of the 400 respondents had seen girls drop out of school sport because of concerns about the kit they had to wear, citing reasons from impracticability to hypersexualization. Interestingly, Tess's research arose from her observations that in men's hockey, players wear shirts and shorts, but in women's hockey, players wear vests and skirts. She asked why, and the only answer people could muster was 'because it's always been like that'. A research study in Australia showed that girls were significantly more active at school break times when wearing their sports uniform compared with their regular school uniform, yet boys' activity levels were the same regardless of what uniform they wore.[8] The difference? The girls' school uniform was a skirt, but their sports uniform was a pair of shorts. Girls were more active when they wore shorts throughout the day than when they were made to wear skirts. When you put it like this, it feels like a really simple solution, doesn't it? But those deeply entrenched traditions to do with uniforms seem to still take priority over a physical inactivity crisis in girls. Things need to change!

To truly belong

We believe that if women can't immerse themselves fully into their fitness and sports activities, as women, then they simply don't truly belong there. Belonging doesn't mean changing who we are to fit in; it's about being exactly who we are and having that fully acknowledged and supported. For too long, in sport, women have had to fit into a men's system that often doesn't consider who women truly are. Women have periods and menstrual cycles, they may use hormonal contraception, they have breasts, they are far more likely to have pelvic floor dysfunction and they have a much higher risk of injury. We often manage emotions, derive confidence and are motivated differently from men. But for a long time, all these things have been regularly hidden, unspoken or dismissed in sport and exercise. It's as though we aren't allowed to show up as women; we have to leave some of the female parts of ourselves at the door. Sometimes, the reasons we do this are inside our heads, but often they're planted there without our permission by society's attitudes, values, beliefs and behaviours. And sometimes, no matter how much we want, or need, to bring our female body into focus, our efforts are dismissed or met with sheer embarrassment. When it comes to being a woman trying to be fit and healthy, we cannot overlook how we are surreptitiously affected by society's attitudes and beliefs about women, women's bodies and women's health.

We started this book with the story of Kathrine Switzer, the first woman to officially run the Boston Marathon, before women were allowed to enter the race. If as recently as 1967 society believed that running a marathon was too great a feat for a woman's body, then is it any wonder that a lack of understanding about women's bodies and exercise still exists, and that instead of realizing its unlimited potential, a woman's body often becomes a barrier to wellness and fitness? Every woman is entitled to a long, happy and healthy relationship with physical activity and movement throughout all stages of her life. Our health is fundamentally supported by our fitness – all the research we have on being physically active shows that it benefits us physically and emotionally – but many women aren't exercising across their lifespan because they don't have the body literacy, confidence or support to enable them to.[9]

When a woman's breast size is the reason she gives for not getting back to netball, a game she loved when she was younger, or when a PE teacher accepts another note about a girl not being able to do sports today because she's on her period, it's not about the bra or the bleed. It's about the entire ecosystem that surrounds these topics. It's the lack of knowledge about the right bra, or that exercise can be good for alleviating period pain. The lack of knowledge comes from the belief that these topics should remain taboo and don't deserve to be part of every woman's education. The lack of education means that while we might know what's to be expected, such as period pain, we might not know what's abnormal, such as period pain that's so intense that it interferes with your daily life. The lack of training specific to women's bodies in qualifications to treat, teach or train girls and women doesn't help, nor does the fact that women don't tend to share their experiences of their bodies freely, to help each generation learn from the last. The lack of research specific to women's bodies means that there often isn't even a solution to some issues, or that accessing the solution can be hard or expensive. The centuries of women's pain and suffering not being taken seriously, with study after study showing that women consistently don't have their pain treated adequately by healthcare professionals, must now change. It's never just about the bra or the bleed. It's about the culture that has existed around women's bodies – and still does.

So how do we change that? It's a big job, to create cultural shifts around such deeply entrenched attitudes and beliefs. Shame and judgement often accompany the topics we've covered in this book. Any one of you reading this will have, at some point, been labelled too fat, too weak or too emotional for sport. You might have been wolf-whistled or sexually harassed as you went on your training run. Perhaps you've felt out of place because you're 'too muscly'. Maybe you've felt intimidated in the weight-lifting section of your gym by the men dominating the space, or you've felt second-class compared to the men at your sports club. These messages are all around us, explicitly or implicitly, from peers, teachers, parents, coaches, television and social media.

But change is happening – slowly, but it's happening. And it's happening because people are speaking up, people are having conversations – honest and vulnerable discussions. Take Jazmin Sawyers, the long jumper who, after she had yet another bout of debilitating period pain at the Rio Olympics, felt the need to speak out about how it wrecked her chances of success on the biggest platform of her life, all because she felt like it was something she had to just put up with, rather than be seen as fragile in her high-performing environment.[10] Or Holly Hill, a rower whose breast pain was so bad it stopped her from training at certain times of the month, and for a long time she had a physio taping up her chest because she didn't know that a well-fitting bra could be her answer. Or Fi Tomas, a reporter for the *Telegraph* who is dedicated to bringing women's health in sport into the mainstream conversation, covering topics such as endometriosis, the pill, pelvic floor dysfunction and women's kit in sport in her articles. Or the This Girl Can campaign showing Hannah Johnson with period pain getting up and out to the gym, with a peek of a tampon string in the advert for good measure. Or Davina McCall, pushing the menopause on to prime-time television in the UK with her documentaries and book entitled *Menopausing*.[11] The more people hear the words, the more they hear the conversations, and the more they see the appetite from women to know more, the more information and discussion about our female body – in terms of its function and capability (rather than its aesthetics and sex appeal) – will be brought out of the shadows, to the benefit of everyone.

What we can do, as individuals, as women, as parents of girls, as managers, peers and friends of women, is to stop the judgement – of ourselves and of others. As many as 85% of people can remember a shaming experience at school that affects their experiences through the rest of their life.[12] One comment from a PE teacher or coach can affect an individual's confidence, self-belief and motivation to do sport for the rest of their life. When we want to support girls and women to fulfil their potential, we have to be mindful of the words we use and the judgement those words can impart. This is especially important because women are far more likely than men to respond to these words with a self-critical inner voice. In girls more than boys, sport highlights insecurities about body image and the fear of what people think of how they look or perform. Judgement fuels those insecurities.

Wouldn't it be incredible to exist in a world where women are free to discuss female-specific challenges without the fear of being labelled weak or hormonal? Encouraging women to discuss period problems, stress incontinence, and the difficulty in finding the right sports bra will enable us all to find others who have overcome similar issues, or to be pointed to the best support before these challenges become the reason we repeatedly opt out of doing exercise or, worse still, stop completely. In our experience, women are often very happy to talk with one another about these topics, given the opportunity. But it often takes someone to take the lead, create the space, give them permission to share.

Let's be more open in sharing our stories, first with other women, and also with the people who support them. We have to stop smuggling tampons up our sleeve or euphemizing periods or accepting that wetting ourselves is a natural part of doing sport as a woman. We need to work together, raising our voices about our bodies, getting curious about what's normal and what's not, sharing what works and what doesn't.

We know it isn't always easy to have conversations about topics that seem private and personal. That's why, at The Well HQ, we developed the ACT BRAVER guidelines, to help people open up the conversation around women's bodies and exercise. Whether you're an active woman wanting to share your story to inspire others, or someone who treats, trains or teaches active women, we hope these guidelines might help you find the boundaries and the confidence you need to challenge the status quo, to speak up, speak out or support others.

ACT BRAVER

Avoid euphemisms, but don't avoid the topics!

Use the right words rather than skirting around the subject with air quotes. If you're talking about periods, say periods. If you need to say vagina, say vagina. The thing with words is that the embarrassment or awkwardness we associate with them are just connections in our brain. Your experiences of that word and the response it got, the way society uses it and responds to it, have all programmed your brain to respond to that word in a certain way. The more we use the right words, the more we can rewire our brains out of the squeamishness we've developed around them.

Confident and courageous

Make sure you arm yourself with the information you need to be confident in these conversations. We've found that one of the biggest barriers to these important conversations is lack of confidence. When women lack confidence in their own or someone else's knowledge, and are therefore uncomfortable talking about these topics, it usually equals permanent avoidance of any discussion.

Travel compassionately

Everyone is coming to these topics from their own set of experiences, values and biases. Meet them there and bring them on a journey with you. Some people will never have said the word 'period' out loud before. Some people will have been taught different words for things. No one will know what *your* period pain feels like. Be generous and patient with others' starting points.

Boundaries

Create boundaries around the topics you want to talk about. If you want to talk to your personal trainer about breast pain, be clear that you want to chat about it because it's affecting the exercise you can do on certain days. Know that it's OK to say when there's information you don't want to share, or to check if someone else is comfortable having a chat about what you want to discuss.

Resentment

Sometimes people will resent what you are saying, in a #notallmen/teachers/doctors, sort of way. If someone's offence gives them an excuse to sit on the sidelines, or to avoid important conversations, then they are part of the problem. Try to use language and tone that imply that no one is to blame for the current predicament and all of us are responsible for forging a path forward. Also be prepared to come across people who resent the fact that if we succeed in making life better for women, then they will have been dealt a worse hand than future generations. It's not a great perspective, but trust us when we say, it's out there.

Across the lifespan

Women's bodies change across our life stages. Some life stages are inevitable for women, like puberty and menopause, and some are possible but not certain, like pregnancy and childbirth. Don't apply a one-size-fits-all approach to your body across your life, and don't expect your experience of your body to remain consistent through the years.

Vault

All the topics we cover in this book could be private and personal for someone. It is a privilege to be trusted with other people's experiences and stories. When talking about women's health issues, you need to be clear about how important this confidentiality is to you, to ensure that others don't share information and experiences that are not theirs to share.

Empower, don't impose

Empowering people is harder than just imposing your opinion or a solution on them. Every woman's experience of her body is different, and often your experience, what worked for you, or what is normal for you, will be different from someone else's experience and solutions. Try to stay curious, ask questions, really listen to the answers, and show empathy – connect to how someone feels about something, rather than just trying to fix the situation altogether.

Remove judgement

Create conversations and spaces where women feel safe to talk about their bodies and how they feel about them, without fear of judgement, criticism or dismissal. Try to be supportive of perception as well as reality – a woman might have a fear of leaking urine that stops her from exercising, and that experience is as important as someone who actually does leak when they move. Support others who have been judged, criticized or dismissed to develop the confidence to go back again and ask for help, or to help someone else understand the impact of their actions or words.

With this book we hope to set a new, higher standard for what we feel every active woman should know. We know it will take time for everyone to feel comfortable and confident with some of these topics, and we're OK with that because we're sick of being invisible and witnessing women compromising their health, well-being and performance because their bodies and their needs aren't being acknowledged in sport and exercise.

We're optimistic about how the future of women's sport is going to look and feel. We're no longer willing to accept that sport is a system built for men. Women participate too, and we belong. We believe that for women to have an equal right to sport and exercise we must look at fitness and performance through a female filter, considering all the female-specific factors that we've covered in this book, so that, as active women, we can truly get the best out of ourselves, whatever our ambitions are in sport, from personal achievements to podium performance. Here's to a revolution where we unleash the power of our female bodies.

Who We Are

Dr Emma Ross: The Scientist

If I were to use one word to describe myself, it would be 'disruptive'. I used to use words like 'passionate' and 'ambitious', but I've settled on disruptive. And not in the same way my two small children can be disruptive: loud and chaotic, breaking silences with shrieks and roars. An innermost kind of disruptive. On the outside, I'm smiley, I love to laugh and sing and joke. But somewhere deep within my DNA is a relentlessly restless soul with a mind to disrupt systems and ideas, to challenge the status quo, to be intolerant of inequality, and to take action to make things better. When I get invited to talk to the graduating classes at the universities I used to work at, my favourite thing to say is 'Always ask for forgiveness, never permission.'

After I completed my PhD in exercise neurophysiology, I became a lecturer and research scientist in the field of sport and exercise science. My early research projects used brain stimulation to study how the brain sends signals to our muscles. I used magnetic brain-stimulation equipment about the size of a couple of microwaves. It lived in the research laboratory and had only ever been used there. But real life doesn't happen in a laboratory, and when I was offered the chance to join a research trip to Mount Everest to study the effects of low oxygen on the brain, I became the first person in the world to take this magnetic-stimulation equipment out of the lab. And not just out of the lab, but up the world's tallest mountain on the side of a yak. Disruptive science.

After I'd been lecturing and researching for about a decade, I was approached to take a role at the English Institute of Sport (EIS) as the Head of Physiology. The EIS is the science and medicine arm of the UK's Olympic and Paralympic system, where sports scientists, doctors and physiotherapists support the elite coaches and athletes in their pursuit of audacious sporting goals. I led the sports scientist team throughout the Rio and Tokyo Olympic cycles.

In 2016 I was given a project at work that would change the course of my life. I was asked to explore whether we supported female athletes within the high-performance sports system. It turned out that we didn't and there is lots more we can do.

The next five years would be spent understanding what's important to consider in terms of supporting women's health, well-being and performance in sport, and then teaching coaches, athletes, sports scientists and anyone else who would listen. I uncovered huge gaps in our knowledge and understanding of the female body in sport and set about trying to change that. The reason that project changed my life is because it made me realize that this was it – this was the impact I wanted to have in the world. In my own small way, I wanted to disrupt everything we have ever accepted or settled for when it comes to caring for and supporting women in sport.

I left my role at the EIS in 2020 to make sure that the reach of my work extended out of elite sport and touched all girls and women who wanted to be active, fit and healthy. And that's what brought me to The Well HQ with Baz and Bella. In 2021 I was awarded the *Sunday Times* Sportswomen of the Year Changemaker Award for my work supporting girls and women in sport.

Outside of work, I am mum to two brilliant children, a son and a daughter, who, after listening to all my online presentations during the home-working lockdown in 2020 and 2021, know more about women's bodies than most people! Having been sporty in my younger days, competing at Twickenham while playing university rugby, and completing an Ironman triathlon and a number of ultra-endurance races in my twenties and thirties, I would now describe myself as active, using physical activity like running, cycling and walking for my mental well-being as well as my physical health. Like many other women, I am just getting to grips with how to get the best out of my midlife body.

Baz Moffat: The Coach

What I know about women's health and well-being is neither revolutionary nor clever. It's fundamental knowledge that I believe every woman should have access to. Knowledge is power, and that power is something that I'm passionate about sharing.

From young adult to older years: the journey of a woman is often complicated and sometimes daunting – mine certainly has been. I left university, became an elite athlete, started my own business as a women's health-and-fitness coach, and then became a mother of two children. The diverse and seemingly unconnected steps on my journey have brought me to the opportunity to create The Well HQ with Bella and Emma.

For as long as I can remember, I've been mad about sport. I wanted to be like the girl I knew at school who played squash for Yorkshire, and dreamed of the day when I would have my own tracksuit with 'Yorkshire' emblazoned on the back. I did compete in athletics at county level, yet went no further. I then found rowing when I was twenty-two years old, which was a major shift in my life path because it was only then that I saw that my childhood dream was possible.

The training was relentless, unlike anything I'd known before, but I absolutely loved it. Three years after picking up a set of oars, I'd made it on to the Great Britain squad, and what followed was a life of eat, sleep, row, repeat. Training camps, endless ergo sessions (that's a rowing machine, to the uninitiated), weights, tests to assess my fitness, hundreds of kilometres on the water each week – I was constantly poised on the edge of illness, injury and exhaustion, but I loved it.

In a way, it was a simple life – everything I did was about the boat and what I could do to make it go faster. This mind-over-matter approach was a performance mentality that got me on to the team, into the boat, and on to the podium. It pushed my body to do things that nobody believed it could or should do. I was a machine and this attitude came pretty easily to me. But I now know that there were signs that this approach was neither sustainable nor healthy.

Fast forward six years and I'd retired from rowing and was pregnant with my eldest son. The pregnancy was great, and my body was behaving brilliantly. It really didn't seem to require much effort on my part. And, because of this and my background as an athlete, I naively assumed that I'd also nail the birth . . . Big mistake!

Somehow, I'd missed out a huge piece of the jigsaw – birth is not a fitness test that you can just push through, it's a completely involuntary process that you can't control. The expectation-versus-reality of my actual birthing experience left me in a state of shock and the aftermath had me questioning who I was. Without anyone to talk to and, assuming it was something everyone felt, I put my head down and cracked on with life. It took me years to bounce back.

I was petrified during my second pregnancy because I assumed I wouldn't be able to have a natural birth. I was all up for drugs to help me through it until my midwife planted the seed about home births. She suggested that I could go into labour feeling safe, private and unobserved. This would have been too 'woo woo' for me the first time around. I didn't end up having the opportunity for a home birth, but because I'd shifted my mind-set towards that option, I connected with my body during childbirth. As my body went deeper and deeper into labour, I gradually let go, and as my body took over, I felt better and better. Every time I had a contraction, I was one step closer to meeting my baby and it was the most empowering and beautiful experience of my life. That labour and delivery blows any other achievement I've had out of the water. It was a true connection on every level, which delivered not only my baby, but also a better version of myself.

There's an honesty and integrity about being so connected with your body. It was an extreme and once-in-a-lifetime experience. It's not something that every woman will have the privilege of experiencing, but I believe I did for an important reason, which was to show me the true power of being a woman. I realize now that every cell in my body knows how to connect. I know first-hand that we can fully, deeply engage and believe in ourselves. I know my experiences have pointed me here to do more, to go deeper with women, to help them connect, to support their education and empowerment, and ultimately to help them identify the strength they have within.

What I do today isn't just about helping women strengthen, relax and coordinate muscles and ligaments in their pelvis; the impact of this work is far-reaching – beyond the bladder, bowel and uterus. When women improve their pelvic floor function, it also builds confidence in their ability to improve their health, which is such an empowering experience.

What I love about both Dr Emma and Dr Bella is that we all share this fundamental belief that every woman is different and that, given the right education and support, girls and women are the ones who are best placed to make the right decisions about their health, and that's something that we're on a mission to make possible.

Dr Bella Smith: The Doctor

Throughout my career as a doctor, I've been surprised and frustrated to hear heartbreaking stories of women who've endured embarrassment and shame surrounding their health and suffered in silence. The stigma that surrounds women's health and well-being persists. It's my ambition to reduce health inequalities and to arm women with the information they need to be the best ambassadors for their own wellness.

From a very young age, I knew that I wanted to be a doctor, inspired by my wonderful mum, who was a nurse for over fifty years. She loved every minute of her job and retired just before the Covid-19 lockdown in 2020. Growing up, I watched her thrive as a nurse. She is brilliantly practical, ridiculously hard-working and, most importantly, has a naughty sense of humour – vital in the medical profession. She taught me the facts of life without my realizing it, and as a result, I was never embarrassed talking about anything and friends often gravitated to me for advice.

When I was fourteen, I recall a school friend being mortified when she realized her period had leaked through her underwear and the spotting was visible on the back of her school skirt. Without hesitation, I took her bloodied skirt and scrubbed it clean before drying it and giving it back to her, adding that there was nothing to be ashamed of. The truth is that this can and does happen to all women at some point in our lives. It made a lasting impression on me and reinforced my desire to be a doctor.

Fast forward twenty-five years and I'm a local doctor seeing hundreds of women weekly in my surgery to discuss all their health needs. I'm also incredibly proud to be an ambassador for The Eve Appeal, a leading UK gynaecological cancer charity, where we talk openly about all aspects of women's health issues while raising funds for, and awareness of, gynaecological cancers.

Having not been particularly sporty in my youth, I've fallen in love with exercise as an adult. We can and should all be active for the sake of physical and mental health. There is no right or wrong way to exercise. The key is to find something you love and enjoy it, and then you're more likely to keep doing it.

When I met Baz and Emma, I realized that, with our different backgrounds, experiences and expertise, and as clichéd as it sounds, we were far greater than the sum of our parts. And that's why we set up The Well HQ. We want to leave a legacy, we want to change the system, and we want to inform and empower you to know your body, strip away the shame and help you become fitter, healthier and happier.

Acknowledgements

This book wouldn't have been possible without many, many wonderful people. We would all like to thank:

Charlotte, our agent. When we were about to hit the self-publish button, you gave us the confidence to believe that we could find a bigger platform for the book, without ever having read a word of it. When we saw your 'Feminist' bag hanging on your chair during our first Zoom call, I think we all knew this was the start of something brilliant! Your patience and quiet resolve has made the journey far less stressful, and your support has allowed us to navigate the foreign world of publishing while staying true to our voice and what we wanted to say.

The team at Transworld, from our editor Steph Duncan and copy-editor Alex Newby to the design, production, publicity, marketing and sales teams, who all played their part in bringing this book to you. The time and energy you put into shaping the final edits were so valuable, and we especially appreciated the extra mile you went to in making sure the science was decoded enough to make sense to everyone, and not just people in lab coats.

Patti, who believed in us from day dot. Who worked with our original idea and our very early drafts. Who told us we'd written three books' worth of content, but didn't make us feel daunted by the prospect of cutting and culling it down to the finished version. Who noticed when we were on our knees but putting on a brave face. Without you, this project would never have got off the ground, and would never had survived that dismal first year of lockdown madness. We will always remember our time with you every Thursday afternoon, before picking up the kids, with such fondness. You expertly guided us through the writing process and allowed us to find our voice.

Everyone at The Well HQ – a team that steps up and jumps right in. Our geography spans from the white cliffs of Sussex to the lowlands of Latvia, and our start-up mentality usually means chaos is ensuing at any moment, but we've created something really special together and we are so grateful that you have joined us in the revolution! Jemima, Ally and Laura, Juliette, Sophie, Danielle and Ashley, if we are the team she needs, then you are the team we need!

Our community of amazing women and men – some athletes, some active women, some parents of daughters, some teachers, some coaches, physios, doctors, researchers. You are a brilliant bunch, who are willing to be some of the first to challenge the status quo for women in sport and fitness. Writing this book and launching our business during Covid felt like we were in a bubble a lot of the time and we often didn't even know if anybody was listening. But publishing this book has made us realize that there's a whole world out there ready to make some big changes. Without you all messaging and talking to us, we might have lost our momentum. Thank you and keep it up.

Original investors, who believed in us before we even started. And Zoe, Liz, Carla, Imogen, Maria, Lindsay, Suzie and Hen – thank you for getting us going. Investing in female founders, setting up a business for females, goes against the grain, and without you none of what's happening right now would be happening! We hope we continue to make you proud and pleased to be an integral part of our journey.

From Emma

About two months before we handed over the final draft of the book to the publishing team, my dad died suddenly. He was my biggest fan, and it makes me so sad to think that he won't be the first one in the queue at the bookstore, buying up the place and telling his golf buddies all about it. I miss you so much, Dad, but when I think about where I am now, how unafraid I have been to just go for things, in work and in life, I owe every bit of that attitude to you. And I am so certain about living my life like that because you were always there as a cornerstone of unconditional love. When I wanted to leave my stable and sought-after job to start a business with Baz and Bella, instead of offering sensible advice you were literally the wind beneath my wings. The email you wrote, shortly before you left us, has kept me going through the darkest of times, because I know you would be so proud to see this book finally out in the world: 'There is a brave new world out there to be created, and it makes Mum and I so proud that you are at the forefront of this change. The world's your oyster, my darling. Go grab it!!!'

To Mum: I don't think there is a kinder, more generous soul on this earth than you. All that I have done, pursued and achieved is because I had your love and support, and because you have so seamlessly extended that love and support to the kids. I love you million, squillions.

To Fraz and Georgie: from near or far, you are always so supportive of me. I hope, in time, the girls love this book, and learn from it to love themselves, to be themselves and maybe even be inspired to become the next architects of a brighter future for women and girls.

To my crew: what would I do without you? You have been such brilliant cheerleaders as we launched The Well HQ, a shoulder to cry on (too many times to count!), but oh so many laughs, too. You are my marble-jar friends and I will love you always.

To Charlotte, my bestie: I don't think either of us could have predicted what the road ahead would hold, as we walked into St Luke's nearly two and a half decades ago, but I know everything that's happened has been made brighter because of our friendship.

To Sophie B: you are a rock star. I feel so lucky that our girls' friendship brought us together, and I am so grateful for all the times you've helped out when I didn't quite know what the f@ck was going on in my life! And for the shared love of GD. This book was a hard thing, and I did it!

To my gorgeous family: Ash, you have taught me so much that has ended up woven through the pages of this book. Thank you for giving me the time and space I needed to write and the opportunity to vent about the process. Thank you for being steadfast in your support since Dad died – I don't think I would have had the headspace to finish this book if you hadn't sat with me in my grief so compassionately. To Bodhi and Brooke: never change – I love all that you are. You are caring, curious, and brilliant little people and I am so proud to be your mummy. I hope this book, and The Well HQ, goes to show you what's possible when you find your purpose, and that you don't have to put up with things because they have always been done that way. I can't wait to see what wonderful marks you make on this world.

And finally to Baz and Bella: Baz, I'm so glad I eventually responded to your stalker-ish email! From the moment I met you, I knew you would change the world one day. I am so glad we get to be your co-pilots! Thank you for going all-in with me, for making work not feel like work, and for coaching me when I've lost the plot. Bella, your smile brightens everyone's day! While we were writing this book, you were also a local doctor dealing with Covid, and you not only kept going, but helped us launch the business – you are amazing! Thank you for always checking in, and for being so positive about this book. Ladies, we did it!

From Baz

Thanks to Emma and Bella. Thank you, Emma, for providing the wine for our writing retreats, but more importantly for never compromising on this book. From start to finish, you've been all-in. I always remember the first-draft chapters you wrote – I couldn't stop reading them, and it was a defining moment when I realized what potential we had. Digging deep to be positive, even when we're all done, is not easy, but through this process we've brought the best out of each other and created something that I'd never have been able to accomplish alone. Bella, thank you for being so positive and upbeat over the past three years. Having your medical knowledge has made sure that this book holds its ground in a space which is easy to 'waffle' through. You're so easy to work with and there for us whenever any of us needs to laugh, cry or have a cheer!

Christine Bird and Jenny Burrell, you probably don't know this, but you were both the women that got me out of my post-natal slump six years ago and gave me the belief in myself to start working in women's health. Thank you for showing me the way.

To my friends – who have already bought loads of copies of this book! But who also checked in on me and have been really interested for a really long time. Clare, Bumble, Rosie, Lynne, Jess, Alice, Tash, Carla and Ally – thank you.

To my family – to Tony, for giving me the space I needed to get the writing done; to my boys – for not caring less about this book, which at times has been my everything; to my parents, for setting me up to know that I could do whatever I wanted to achieve; and to Zem, who I know is my biggest fan.

From Bella

Thank you, Baz, for being the best ring-leader and engine behind The Well HQ, who keeps us all going. Without your organizing, inspiration and passion, we would not have all got together and would not be where we are today.

Emma, thank you for being amazing. Not only are you one of the most inspiring, hard-working, knowledgeable, clever people I have ever met, you are also brave and courageous, and have continued to work on, even when faced with personal tragedy.

To Graham, Chloe and Jamie: thank you to my husband and children. My gorgeous, supportive, wonderful little 'Team Smith' that is my everything and my reason for being.

To my parents, Jonnie and Migs, and my big sister Jen, for listening to me, encouraging and being there always. And thank you for helping with all the childcare!!!

To doctor colleagues: Dr Sid and Dr Anna, and all the staff in my surgery, have been so supportive while writing this book. Being a doctor is tough at the best of times, but we are a strong team and I am so grateful to work with such awesome people.

To Georgie Dickins, thank you for being so incredibly supportive and for believing I can reach for the stars.

To all my friends and family who are always there for that quick chat, for that essential run after work or that early-morning cycle, and often for that very-needed glass of wine: thank you all for your love, moral support and also for buying the book and shouting about it on our behalf. xxx

Notes on Sources

1: Mind the Gaps

1   Tejas Kotecha, 'Kathrine Switzer: First woman to officially run Boston Marathon on the iconic moment she was attacked by the race organiser', Sky Sports, https://www.skysports.com/more-sports/athletics/news/29175/12475824/kathrine-switzer-first-woman-to-officially-run-boston-marathon-on-the-iconic-moment-she-was-attacked-by-the-race-organiser

2   Kathrine Switzer, *Marathon Woman* (Carroll & Graf, 2007).

3   Emma S. Cowley, Alyssa A. Olenick, Kelly L. McNulty et al., ' "Invisible sportswomen": the sex data gap in sport and exercise science research', *Women in Sport and Physical Activity Journal*, 29: 2 (2021), pp. 146–51: https://journals.humankinetics.com/view/journals/wspaj/29/2/article-p146.xml

4   Min Zhao, Sreenivas P. Veeranki, Costan G. Magnussen et al., 'Recommended physical activity and all cause and cause specific mortality in US adults: prospective cohort study', *BMJ*: https://www.bmj.com/content/370/bmj.m2031

5   Stephen W. Farrell, Shannon J. Fitzgerald, Paul A. McAuley et al., 'Cardiorespiratory fitness, adiposity, and all-cause mortality in women', *Medicine and Science in Sports and Exercise*, 42: 11 (2010), pp. 2006–12: doi: 10.1249/MSS.0b013e3181df12bf. PMID: 20351588

6   James Clear, *Atomic Habits* (Random House Business, 2018), p. 27.

7   'Better for Women', Royal College of Obstetricians and Gynaecologists, December 2019: https://www.rcog.org.uk/media/h3smwohw/better-for-women-full-report.pdf

8   Leanne Norman and Jamie French, 'Understanding how high performance women athletes experience the coach–athlete relationship', *International Journal of Coaching Science*, 7: 1 (2013), pp. 3–24: https://www.semanticscholar.org/paper/Understanding-how-High-Performance-Women-Athletes-Norman-French/12ad213a4973efae47b72e432440ia4ade95cbf5

9   Joseph T. Costello, François Bieuzen and Chris M. Bleakley, 'Where are all the female participants in sports and exercise medicine science research?', *European Journal of Sport Science*, 14: 8 (2014), pp. 847–51: https://www.tandfonline.com/doi/abs/10.1080/17461391.2014.911354

10   Emma S. Cowley et al., 'Invisible Sportswomen'.

11   Caroline Criado Perez, *Invisible Women: Exposing Data Bias in a World Designed for Men* (Chatto & Windus, 2019), p. 204.

12   Kelly Lee McNulty, Kirsty Jane Elliot-Sale, Eimear Dolan et al., 'The effects of menstrual cycle phase on exercise performance in eumenorrheic women: a systematic review and meta-analysis', *Sports Medicine*, 50: 10 (2020), pp. 1813–27: https://pubmed.ncbi.nlm.nih.gov/32661839/

13   Eunsook Sung, Ahreum Han, Tino Hinrichs et al., 'Effects of follicular versus luteal phase-based strength training in young women', *SpringerPlus*, 3 (2014), p. 668: https://www.ncbi.nlm.nih.gov/pmc/articles/PMC4236309/

14   Lawrence W. Green, Judith M. Ottoson, César García et al., 'Diffusion theory and knowledge dissemination, utilization, and integration in public health', *Annual Review of Public Health*, 30 (2009), pp. 151–74: https://pubmed.ncbi.nlm.nih.gov/19705558/

15   Marsa Daniel and Sam Moore, 'Why isn't women's-specific training more widespread within sport? Bridging the gap between research and applied practice', presentation at the Female Athlete Conference, Boston Children's Hospital, 10 June 2021.

2: Health and Fitness Through a Female Filter

1   Conor Stewart, 'Contraceptive use among women in England 2019/20', *Statista*, September 2021: https://www.statista.com/statistics/573210/contraceptive-use-among-women-by-type-and-age-in-england/

2   Jenny Burbage, Michelle Norris, Brogan Horler et al., 'Breast health and the exercising female' in Jacky Forsyth and Claire-Marie Roberts, eds., *The Exercising Female: Science and its Application* (Routledge, 2019).

3   Atefeh Omrani, Joanna Wakefield-Scurr, Jenny Smith et al., 'Breast education improves adolescent girls' breast knowledge, attitudes to breasts and engagement with positive breast habits', *Frontiers in Public Health*, 8: 591927 (2020): https://www.frontiersin.org/article/10.3389/fpubh.2020.591927

4   Celeste E. Coltman, Julie R. Steele and Deirdre E. McGhee, 'Does breast size affect how women participate in physical activity?', *Journal of Science and Medicine in Sport*, 22: 3 (2019), pp. 324–9: https://www.jsams.org/article/S1440-2440(18)30875-2/fulltext

5   Joanne L. Parsons, Stephanie E. Coen and Sheree Bekker, 'Anterior cruciate ligament injury: towards a gendered environmental approach', *British Journal of Sports Medicine*, 55 (2021), pp. 984–90: https://bjsm.bmj.com/content/55/17/984

6   Jennifer Moriatis Wolf, Lisa K. Cannada, Ann Van Heest et al., 'Male and female differences in musculoskeletal disease', *Journal of the American Academy of Orthopaedic Surgeons*, 23: 6 (2015), pp. 339–47: https://www.researchgate.net/publication/277079715_Male_and_Female_Differences_in_Musculoskeletal_Disease

7   Kay M. Crossley, Brooke E. Patterson, Adam G. Culvenor et al., 'Making football safer for women: a systematic review and meta-analysis of injury prevention programmes in 11 773 female football (soccer) players', *British Journal of Sports Medicine*, 54 (2020), pp. 1089–98: https://bjsm.bmj.com/content/54/18/1089

8   Throughout this book, when we refer to inflammation, we mean systemic, or full body inflammation. Your immune system is activated when your body recognizes anything that is foreign – such as an invading microbe or plant pollen. This often triggers a process called inflammation. Intermittent bouts of inflammation directed at truly threatening invaders are important to protect your health. However, sometimes inflammation persists even when you are not threatened by a foreign invader. That's when inflammation can become detrimental to our health. Many major diseases that plague us including cancer, heart disease, diabetes, arthritis, depression and Alzheimer's have been linked to chronic inflammation, and menstrual cycle and perimenopausal symptoms have been shown to be made worse in the presence of inflammation.

9   Lara Briden, *Hormone Repair Manual: Every Woman's Guide to Healthy Hormones* (CreateSpace Independent Publishing Platform, 2017), p. 198.

3: Mastering Your Menstrual Cycle

1   'Better for Women', Royal College of Obstetricians and Gynaecologists, December 2019: https://www.rcog.org.uk/better-for-women

2   'Exercise to feel better during your period, new global study shows', Strava Press, 25 March 2019: https://blog.strava.com/press/exercise-to-feel-better-during-your-period-new-global-study-shows/

3   Anna Druet and Lisa Kennelly, 'Is period slang ever useful?', *Clue*, 20 September 2017: https://helloclue.com/articles/culture/is-period-slang-ever-useful

4   Eamonn Flanagan, 'The gameday primer: principles and practices', *Blk Box*, 19 September 2019: https://www.blkboxfitness.com/blogs/education/the-gameday-primer-principles-and-practices

5   American College of Obstetricians and Gynecologists, 'Menstruation in girls and adolescents: using the menstrual cycle as a vital sign', *Committee Opinion*, 651 (2015): https://www.acog.org/clinical/clinical-guidance/committee-opinion/articles/2015/12/menstruation-in-girls-and-adolescents-using-the-menstrual-cycle-as-a-vital-sign

6   Nathan Brott and Jacqueline Le, 'Mittelschmerz', *StatPearls*, 8 May 2022: https://www.ncbi.nlm.nih.gov/books/NBK549822/

7   Mayo Clinic staff, 'Menorrhagia (heavy menstrual bleeding)', Mayo Clinic: https://www.mayoclinic.org/diseases-conditions/menorrhagia/symptoms-causes/syc-20352829

8   Such as those from period-product company Dame (https://wearedame.co/pages/impact-reports).

9   Two period swimwear brands currently on the market can be found at www.modibodi.com and www.rubylove.com

10   Such as those at https://fablittlebag.com

11   'Period shame causing plastic pollution: 2.4m tampons flushed down the toilet every day', PHS Group, 10 June 2022: https://www.phs.co.uk/about-phs/expertise-news/period-shame-causing-plastic-pollution/

12   Lauren C. Houghton and Noémie Elhadad, 'Practice note: "If only all women menstruated exactly two weeks ago": interdisciplinary challenges and experiences of capturing hormonal variation across the menstrual cycle', in Chris Bobel, Inga T. Winkler, Breanne Fahs et al., eds., *The Palgrave Handbook of Critical Menstruation Studies* (Palgrave Macmillan, 2020), pp. 725–32.

13   Mohaned Shilaih, Brianna M. Goodale, Lisa Falco et al., 'Modern fertility awareness methods: wrist wearables capture the changes in

temperature associated with the menstrual cycle', *Bioscience Reports*, 38: 6 (2018): https://pubmed.ncbi.nlm.nih.gov/29175999/

14   https://hormonix.com

15   Blair T. Crewther and Christian J. Cook, 'A longitudinal analysis of salivary testosterone concentrations and competitiveness in elite and non-elite women athletes', *Physiology and Behavior*, 188 (2018), pp. 157–61: https://pubmed.ncbi.nlm.nih.gov/29425972/

16   C. J. Cook, L. P. Kilduff and B. T. Crewther, 'Basal and stress-induced salivary testosterone variation across the menstrual cycle and linkage to motivation and muscle power', *Scandinavian Journal of Medicine & Science in Sports*, 28: 4 (2018), pp. 1345–53: https://pubmed.ncbi.nlm. nih.gov/29266410/

17   William C. Krause, Ruben Rodriguez, Bruno Gegenhuber et al., 'Oestrogen engages brain MC4R signalling to drive physical activity in female mice', *Nature*, 599 (2021), pp. 131–5: https://www.nature.com/ articles/s41586-021-04010-3

18   Thomas Buser, 'The impact of the menstrual cycle and hormonal contraceptives on competitiveness', *Journal of Economic Behavior & Organization*, 83: 1 (2012), pp. 1–10: https://www.sciencedirect.com/ science/article/abs/pii/S016726811100151X

19   Esther K. Diekhof, 'Be quick about it. Endogenous estradiol level, menstrual cycle phase and trait impulsiveness predict impulsive choice in the context of reward acquisition', *Hormones and Behavior*, 74 (2015), pp. 186–93: https://www.sciencedirect.com/science/article/ abs/pii/S0018506X1500104X

20   Hadine Joffe, Anouk de Wit, Jamie Coborn et al., 'Impact of estradiol variability and progesterone on mood in perimenopausal women with depressive symptoms', *Journal of Clinical Endocrinology and Metabolism*, 105: 4 (2020), e642–50: https://pubmed.ncbi.nlm.nih. gov/31693131/

21   Katy Vincent, Charlotte J. Stagg, Catherine E. Warnaby et al., ' "Luteal analgesia": progesterone dissociates pain intensity and unpleasantness by influencing emotion regulation networks', *Frontiers in Endocrinology*, 9: 413 (2018): https://www.readcube.com/ articles/10.3389/fendo.2018.00413

22   Haneul Lee, Jerrold Petrofsky, Nirali Shah et al., 'Higher sweating rate and skin blood flow during the luteal phase of the menstrual cycle', *Tohoku Journal of Experimental Medicine*, 234: 2 (2014), pp. 11–22: https://pubmed.ncbi.nlm.nih.gov/25230913/

23 Heidi Danker-Hopfe, Kirsten Roczen and Ute Löwenstein-Wagner, 'Regulation of food intake during the menstrual cycle', *Anthropologischer Anzeiger*, 53: 3 (1995), pp. 231–8: https://www.jstor.org/stable/29540529

24 'Preventative powers of ovulation and progesterone', Centre for Menstrual Cycle and Ovulation Research (October 2014): https://www.cemcor.ubc.ca/resources/preventive-powers-ovulation-and-progesterone

25 Georgie Bruinvels, Esther Goldsmith, Richard Blagrove et al., 'Prevalence and frequency of menstrual cycle symptoms are associated with availability to train and compete: a study of 6812 exercising women recruited using the Strava exercise app', *British Journal of Sports Medicine*, 55: 8 (2021), pp. 438–44: https://bjsm.bmj.com/content/55/8/438

26 Alice McNamara, Rachel Harris and Clare Minahan, 'Menstrual cycle change during Covid-19. Sharing some early results', *British Journal of Sports Medicine* blog, 20 November 2020: https://blogs.bmj.com/bjsm/2020/11/20/menstrual-cycle-change-during-covid-19/

27 Yi-Xin Wang, Mariel Arvizu, Janet W. Rich-Edwards et al., 'Menstrual cycle regularity and length across the reproductive lifespan and risk of premature mortality: prospective cohort study', *BMJ*, 371: 3464 (2020): https://www.bmj.com/content/371/bmj.m3464

28 Jane Marjoribanks, Michelle Proctor, Cindy Farquhar et al., 'Nonsteroidal anti-inflammatory drugs for dysmenorrhoea', *Cochrane Database of Systematic Reviews*, I (2010), CD001751: https://pubmed.ncbi.nlm.nih.gov/20091521/

29 'Heavy periods', NHS: https://www.nhs.uk/conditions/heavy-periods/treatment/

30 Sang-Dol Kim, 'Yoga for menstrual pain in primary dysmenorrhea: a meta-analysis of randomized controlled trials', *Complementary Therapies in Clinical Practice*, 36 (2019), pp. 94–9: https://www.sciencedirect.com/science/article/abs/pii/S1744388119300945?via%3Dihub

31 Tong Liu, Jia-Ni Yu, Bing-Yan Cao et al., 'Acupuncture for primary dysmenorrhea: a meta-analysis of randomized controlled trials', *Alternative Therapies*, 26: 2 (2020), pp. 46–53: https://search.proquest.com/openview/fde7e8a7513853b114a24a65f4182146/1?pq-origsite=gscholar&cbl=32528

32   George A. Eby, 'Zinc treatment prevents dysmenorrhea', *Medical Hypotheses*, 69: 2 (2007), pp. 297–301: https://www.sciencedirect.com/science/article/abs/pii/S0306987706009066?via%3Dihub

33   Fabio Parazzini, Mirella Di Martino and Paolo Pellegrino, 'Magnesium in the gynecological practice: a literature review', *Magnesium Research*, 30: 1 (2017), pp. 1–7: https://pubmed.ncbi.nlm.nih.gov/28392498/

34   Zeev Harel, Frank M. Biro, Renee K. Kottenhahn et al., 'Supplementation with omega-3 polyunsaturated fatty acids in the management of dysmenorrhea in adolescents', *Americal Journal of Obstetrics & Gynecology*, 174: 4 (1996), pp. 1335–8: https://www.ajog.org/article/S0002-9378(96)70681-6/fulltext

35   Lara Briden, 'The inflammation from A1 milk is mind-boggling', *Lara Briden*, 26 November 2021: https://www.larabriden.com/the-inflammation-from-a1-milk-is-mind-boggling/

36   Samira Khayat, Hamed Fanaei, Masoomeh Kheirkhah et al., 'Curcumin attenuates severity of premenstrual syndrome symptoms: a randomized, double-blind, placebo-controlled trial', *Complementary Therapies in Medicine*, 23: 3 (2015), pp. 318–24: https://www.sciencedirect.com/science/article/abs/pii/S096522991500059X

37   Alexandre Vallée and Yves Lecarpentier, 'Curcumin and endometriosis', *International Journal of Molecular Sciences*, 21: 2440 (2020): https://www.mdpi.com/1422-0067/21/7/2440

38   Chooi L. Wong, Cindy Farquhar, Helen Roberts et al., 'Oral contraceptive pill for primary dysmenorrhoea', *Cochrane Database of Systematic Reviews*, 4 (2009), CD002120: https://www.ncbi.nlm.nih.gov/pmc/articles/PMC7154221/#CD002120-bbs2-0031

39   'PMS (premenstrual syndrome)', NHS: https://www.nhs.uk/conditions/pre-menstrual-syndrome/

40   Kimberley Ann Yonkers, Shaughn O'Brien and Elias Eriksson, 'Premenstrual syndrome', *Lancet*, 371: 9619 (2008), pp. 1200–10: https://www.ncbi.nlm.nih.gov/pmc/articles/PMC3118460/

41   'Definitions PMS/PMDD', National Association for Premenstrual Syndromes: https://www.pms.org.uk/about-pms/definitions-pms-pmdd/

42   'About PMS: What is PMS?', National Association for Premenstrual Syndromes: https://www.pms.org.uk/about-pms/

43   John F. Steege and James A. Blumenthal, 'The effects of aerobic exercise on premenstrual symptoms in middle-aged women: a

preliminary study', *Journal of Psychosomatic Research*, 37: 2 (1993), pp. 127–33: https://www.sciencedirect.com/science/article/abs/pii/002239999390079U; Zeinab Samadi, Farzaneh Taghian and Mahboubeh Valiani, 'The effects of 8 weeks of regular aerobic exercise on the symptoms of premenstrual syndrome in non-athlete girls', *Iranian Journal of Nursing and Midwifery Research*, 18: 1 (2013), pp. 14–99: https://pubmed.ncbi.nlm.nih.gov/23983722/

44   A. Steptoe and S. Cox, 'Acute effects of aerobic exercise on mood', *Health Psychology*, 7: 4 (1988), pp. 329–40: https://pubmed.ncbi.nlm.nih.gov/3168978/

45   Sonja Aalbers, Laura Fusar-Poli, Ruth E. Freeman et al., 'Music therapy for depression', *Cochrane Database of Systematic Reviews*, 11: 11 (2017), CD004517: https://pubmed.ncbi.nlm.nih.gov/29144545/

46   Andrea Chisholm, '5 things women need to know about diabetes and their period', *Verywell Health*, 25 July 2022: https://www.verywellhealth.com/diabetes-and-womens-menstrual-cycles-4067212

47   'Prostaglandins', *You and Your Hormones*: https://www.yourhormones.info/hormones/prostaglandins/

48   Semra Kocaoz, Rabiye Cirpan and Arife Zuhal Degirmencioglu, 'The prevalence and impacts [of] heavy menstrual bleeding on anemia, fatigue and quality of life in women of reproductive age', *Pakistan Journal of Medical Sciences*, 35: 2 (2019), pp. 365–70: https://www.ncbi.nlm.nih.gov/pmc/articles/PMC6500811/

49   Georgie Bruinvels, Richard Burden, Nicola Brown et al., 'The prevalence and impact of heavy menstrual bleeding (menorrhagia) in elite and non-elite athletes', *PLOS One*, 11: 2 (2016), e0149881: https://journals.plos.org/plosone/article?id=10.1371/journal.pone.0149881

50   Ibid.

51   Emma Burnett, Jenny White and Joanna Wakefield-Scurr, 'The validity and reliability of a breast pain diary for women with cyclic breast pain', School of Sport, Health & Exercise at the University of Portsmouth at Pain Science in Motion 2015 event: https://researchportal.port.ac.uk/en/publications/the-validity-and-reliability-of-a-breast-pain-diary-for-women-wit

52   D. N. Ader, J. South-Paul, T. Adera et al., 'Cyclical mastalgia: prevalence and associated health and behavioral factors', Journal of Psychosomatic Obstetrics and Gynecology, 22:

2 (2001), pp. 71–6: https://www.tandfonline.com/doi/abs/10.3109/01674820109049956

53 Diana L. Dell, 'Premenstrual syndrome, premenstrual dysphoric disorder, and premenstrual exacerbation of another disorder', *Clinical Obstetrics and Gynecology*, 47: 3 (2004), pp. 568–75: https://journals.lww.com/clinicalobgyn/Citation/2004/09000/Premenstrual_Syndrome,_Premenstrual_Dysphoric.10.aspx

54 G. Allais, Giulia Chiarle, Silvia Sinigaglia et al., 'Menstrual migraine: a review of current and developing pharmacotherapies for women', *Expert Opinion on Pharmacotherapy*, 19: 2 (2018), pp. 123–36: https://www.tandfonline.com/doi/abs/10.1080/14656566.2017.1414182?journalCode=ieop20

55 William E. Whitehead, Lawrence J. Cheskin, Barbara R. Heller et al., 'Evidence for exacerbation of irritable bowel syndrome during menses', *Gastroenterology*, 98: 6 (1990), pp. 1485–9: https://pubmed.ncbi.nlm.nih.gov/2338190/

56 Merry Noel Miller and B. E. Miller, 'Premenstrual exacerbations of mood disorders', *Psychopharmacology Bulletin*, 35: 3 (2001), pp. 135–49: https://pubmed.ncbi.nlm.nih.gov/12397883/

57 Clár McWeeny, 'Premenstrual magnification: mental health conditions and PMS', *Clue*, 11 July 2017: https://helloclue.com/articles/cycle-a-z/mental-health-pms-what-happens-when-mental-health-conditions-coincide-with-pms

58 Sarah Young, 'Endometriosis takes average of eight years to diagnose, new report finds', *Independent*, 19 October 2020: https://www.independent.co.uk/life-style/women/endometriosis-symptoms-diagnosis-support-inquiry-b1152552.html

59 www.verity-pcos.org.uk

60 Lara Briden, 'Treatment for 4 types of PCOS. Treat the cause', *Lara Briden*, 16 May 2014: https://www.larabriden.com/treatment-for-4-types-of-pcos-treat-the-cause/

61 Kelly Lee McNulty, Kirsty Jayne Elliott-Sale, Eimear Dolan et al., 'The effects of menstrual cycle phase on exercise performance in eumenorrheic women: a systematic review and meta-analysis', *Sports Medicine*, 50 (2020), pp. 1813–27: https://pubmed.ncbi.nlm.nih.gov/32661839/

62 Sarah McKay, *Demystifying the Female Brain: A Neuroscientist Explores Health, Hormones and Happiness* (Orion Spring, 2018).

63 Joan M. Eckerson, 'Energy and the nutritional needs of the exercising female', in Jacky Forsyth and Claire-Marie Roberts, eds., *The Exercising Female: Science and its Application* (Routledge, 2018), pp. 44–65.

64 Tanya Oosthuyse and Andrew N. Bosch, 'The effect of the menstrual cycle on exercise metabolism', *Sports Medicine*, 40: 3 (2010), pp. 207–27: https://link.springer.com/article/10.2165/11317090-000000000-00000

65 Melissa M. Markofski and William A. Braun, 'Influence of menstrual cycle on indices of contraction-induced muscle damage', *Journal of Strength and Conditioning Research*, 28: 9 (2014), pp. 2649–56: https://journals.lww.com/nsca-jscr/Fulltext/2014/09000/Influence_of_Menstrual_Cycle_on_Indices_of.31.aspx

66 Lawrence L. Spriet and Martin J. Gibala, 'Nutritional strategies to influence adaptations to training', *Journal of Sports Science*, 22: 1 (2004), pp. 127–41: https://pubmed.ncbi.nlm.nih.gov/14971438/

67 Eunsook Sung, Ahreum Han, Timo Hinrichs et al., 'Effects of follicular versus luteal phase-based strength training in young women', *SpringerPlus*, 3 (2014), p. 668: https://springerplus.springeropen.com/articles/10.1186/2193-1801-3-668

68 Ibid.

69 E. Reis, U. Frick and D. Schmidtbleicher, 'Frequency variations of strength training sessions triggered by the phases of the menstrual cycle', *International Journal of Sports Medicine*, 16: 8 (1995), pp. 545–50: https://www.thieme-connect.de/products/ejournals/abstract/10.1055/s-2007-973052

70 J. S. Volek, C. E. Forsyth and W. J. Kraemer, 'Nutritional aspects of women strength athletes', *British Journal of Sports Medicine*, 40: 9 (2006), pp. 742–8: https://www.ncbi.nlm.nih.gov/pmc/articles/PMC2564387/

71 Stacy T. Sims, *Roar: How to Match Your Food and Fitness to Your Unique Female Physiology for Optimum Performance, Great Health, and a Strong, Lean Body for Life* (Rodale, 2016).

72 Nkechinyere Chidi-Ogbolu and Keith Baar, 'Effect of estrogen on musculoskeletal performance and injury risk', *Frontiers in Physiology*, 9: 1834 (2018): https://www.frontiersin.org/articles/10.3389/fphys.2018.01834/full

73 Noriko Adachi, Koji Nawata, Michio Maeta et al., 'Relationship of the menstrual cycle phase to anterior cruciate ligament injuries in teenaged female athletes', *Archives of Orthopaedic and Trauma Surgery*, 128:

5 (2008), pp. 473–8: https://link.springer.com/article/10.1007/
s00402-007-0461-1

74   James Kolasinski, Emily L. Hinson, Amir P. Divanbeighi Zand et al.,
      'The dynamics of cortical GABA in human motor learning', *Journal
      of Physiology*, 597: 1 (2019), pp. 271–82: https://physoc.onlinelibrary.
      wiley.com/doi/full/10.1113/JP276626

75   Fawaz Alasmari, 'Caffeine induces neurobehavioral effects through
      modulating neurotransmitters', *Saudi Pharmaceutical Journal*, 28: 4
      (2020), pp. 445–51: https://www.sciencedirect.com/science/article/
      pii/S1319016420300359?via%3Dihub

76   Ronan A. Mooney, James P. Coxon, John Cirillo et al., 'Acute aerobic
      exercise modulates primary motor cortex inhibition', *Experimental
      Brain Research*, 234 (2016), pp. 3669–76: https://link.springer.com/
      article/10.1007/s00221-016-4767-5

77   Joel Mason, Glyn Howatson, Ashlyn K. Frazer et al., 'Modulation
      of intracortical inhabitation and excitation in agonist and antagonist
      muscles following acute strength training', *European Journal of Applied
      Physiology and Occupational Physiology*, 119: 10 (2019), pp. 2185–99:
      https://pubmed.ncbi.nlm.nih.gov/31385029/

4: Your Body on Birth Control

1   'Contraceptive Use by Method 2019', United Nations Department
      of Economic and Social Affairs: https://www.un.org/development/
      desa/pd/sites/www.un.org.development.desa.pd/files/files/
      documents/2020/Jan/un_2019_contraceptiveusebymethod_
      databooklet.pdf

2   www.thelowdown.com

3   Mikkel Oxfeldt, Line B. Dalgaard, Astrid A. Jørgensen et al.,
      'Hormonal contraceptive use, menstrual dysfunctions, and self-
      reported side effects in elite athletes in Denmark', *International
      Journal of Sports Physiology and Performance*, 15: 10 (2020), pp. 1377–
      84: https://journals.humankinetics.com/view/journals/ijspp/15/10/
      article-p1377.xml

4   Sarah Graham, 'Is it safe to skip your period on the pill?', *Patient*,
      31 January 2019: https://patient.info/news-and-features/
      is-it-safe-to-skip-your-period-on-the-pill

5   Sarah Hill, *How the Pill Changes Everything: Your Brain on Birth
      Control* (Orion Spring, 2019).

6   Jeffrey F. Peipert, Qiuhong Zhao, Jenifer E. Allsworth et al.,
      'Continuation and satisfaction of reversible contraception', *Obstetrics
      and Gynecology*, 117: 5 (2011), pp. 1105–13: https://www.ncbi.nlm.nih.
      gov/pmc/articles/PMC3548669/

7   Mirena® coil information leaflet, Bayer HealthCare Pharmaceuticals,
      2008: https://www.accessdata.fda.gov/drugsatfda_docs/
      label/2008/021225s019lbl.pdf

8   Eric Wooltorton, 'Medroxyprogesterone acetate (Depo-Provera) and
      bone mineral density loss', *Canadian Medical Association Journal*, 172:
      6 (2005): https://doi.org/10.1503/cmaj.050158

9   'Birth control: benefits beyond pregnancy prevention', *WebMD*,
      14 October 2020: https://www.webmd.com/sex/birth-control/
      other-benefits-birth-control

10   Daniel Martin, Craig Sale, Simon B. Cooper et al., 'Period prevalence
      and perceived side effects of hormonal contraceptive use and the
      menstrual cycle in elite athletes', *International Journal of Sports
      Physiology and Performance*, 13: 7 (2018), pp. 926–32: https://journals.
      humankinetics.com/view/journals/ijspp/13/7/article-p926.xml

11   Johannes Hertel, Johanna König, Georg Homuth et al., 'Evidence
      for stress-like alterations in the HPA-Axis in women taking oral
      contraceptives, *Scientific Reports*, 7 (2017): https://www.nature.com/
      articles/s41598-017-13927-7

12   Agnese Mariotti, 'The effects of chronic stress on health: new insights
      into the molecular mechanisms of brain–body communication', *Future
      Science OA*, 1: 3 (2015), FSO23: https://www.ncbi.nlm.nih.gov/pmc/
      articles/PMC5137920/

13   Brianna Larsen, Amanda Cox, Candice Colbey et al., 'Inflammation
      and oral contraceptive use in female athletes before the Rio Olympic
      Games', *Frontiers in Physiology*, 11: 497 (2020): https://www.
      frontiersin.org/articles/10.3389/fphys.2020.00497/full

14   Sabina Cauci, Cinzia Buligan, Micaela Marangone et al., 'Oxidative
      stress in female athletes using combined oral contraceptives',
      Sports Medicine Open, 2: 40 (2016): https://sportsmedicine-open.
      springeropen.com/articles/10.1186/s40798-016-0064-x

15   Clemens Kirschbaum, Petra Platte, Karl-Martin Pirke et al.,
      'Adrenocortical activation following stressful exercise: further
      evidence for attenuated free cortisol responses in women using oral
      contraceptives', *Stress and Health*, 12: 3 (1996), pp. 137–43: https://

onlinelibrary.wiley.com/doi/abs/10.1002/%28SICI%291099-1700%28199607%2912%3A3%3C137%3A%3AAID-SMI685%3E3.0.CO%3B2-C

16 A. Bonen, F. W. Haynes and T. E. Graham, 'Substrate and hormonal responses to exercise in women using oral contraceptives', *Journal of Applied Physiology*, 70: 5 (1991), pp. 1917–27: https://journals. physiology.org/doi/abs/10.1152/jappl.1991.70.5.1917

17 Anthony C. Hackney and Elizabeth A. Walz, 'Hormonal adaptation and the stress of exercise training: the role of glucocorticoids', *Trends in Sport Sciences*, 20: 4 (2013), pp. 165–71: https://www.ncbi.nlm.nih. gov/pmc/articles/PMC5988244/

18 Chang Woock Lee, Mark A. Newman and Steven E. Riechman, 'Oral contraceptive use impairs muscle gains in young women', *FASEB Journal*, 23: S1 (2009), pp. 955.25–955.25: https://faseb.onlinelibrary. wiley.com/doi/abs/10.1096/fasebj.23.1_supplement.955.25

19 Michael Rosenberg, 'Weight changes with oral contraceptive use and during the menstrual cycle: results of daily measurements', *Contraception*, 58: 6 (1998), pp. 345–9: https://www. contraceptionjournal.org/article/S0010-7824(98)00127-9/fulltext

20 Johannes Hertel et al., 'Evidence for stress-like alterations in the HPA-Axis in women taking oral contraceptives', op. cit.

21 E. Toffol, O. Heikinheimo, P. Koponen et al., 'Hormonal contraception and mental health: results of a population-based study', *Human Reproduction*, 26: 11 (2011), p. 3085–93: https://academic. oup.com/humrep/article/26/11/3085/655818

22 Jill B. Becker, Terry E. Robinson and Kimberly A. Lorenz, 'Sex differences and estrous cycle variations in amphetamine-elicited rotation behavior', *European Journal of Pharmacology*, 80: 1 (1982), pp. 65–72: https://www.sciencedirect.com/science/article/abs/ pii/0014299982901789?via%3Dihub

23 Kirsty J. Elliot-Sale, Kelly L. McNulty, Paul Ansdell et al., 'The effects of oral contraceptives on exercise performance in women: a systematic review and meta-analysis', *Sports Medicine*, 50: 10 (2020), pp. 1785–812: https://pubmed.ncbi.nlm.nih.gov/32666247/

24 Gretchen A. Casazza, Sang-Hoon Suh, Benjamin F. Miller et al., 'Effects of oral contraceptives on peak exercise capacity', *Journal of Applied Physiology*, 93: 5 (2002), pp. 1698–702: https://journals. physiology.org/doi/full/10.1152/japplphysiol.00622.2002

25   C. M. Lebrun, M. A. Petit, D. C. McKenzie et al., 'Decreased maximal aerobic capacity with use of a triphasic oral contraceptive in highly active women: a randomised controlled trial', *British Journal of Sports Medicine*, 37: 4 (2000), pp. 315–20: https://bjsm.bmj.com/content/37/4/315

5: Perfecting Your Pelvic Floor

1   Jennifer M. Wu, Camille P. Vaughan and Patricia S. Goode et al., 'Prevalence and trends of symptomatic pelvic floor disorders in U.S. women', *Obstetrics & Gynecology*, 123: 1 (2014), pp. 141–8: https://pubmed.ncbi.nlm.nih.gov/24463674/

2   Julie Wiebe, 'Dear Canadian Running: are leaks with running "no big deal"?', *Julie Wiebe PT*, 19 August 2019: https://www.juliewiebept.com/dear-canadian-running-are-leaks-with-running-no-big-deal/

3   Kari Bø and Ingrid Elisabeth Nygaard, 'Is physical activity good or bad for the female pelvic floor? A narrative review', *Sports Medicine*, 50: 3 (2020), pp. 471–84: https://link.springer.com/article/10.1007/s40279-019-01243-1

4   Stephanie S. Faubion, Lynne T. Shuster and Adil E. Bharucha, 'Recognition and management of nonrelaxing pelvic floor dysfunction', *Mayo Clinic Proceedings*, 87: 2 (2012): pp. 187–93: https://pubmed.ncbi.nlm.nih.gov/22305030/

5   Ibid.

6   Chi Chiung Grace Chen, Jacob T. Cox, Chloe Yuan et al., 'Knowledge of pelvic floor disorders in women seeking primary care: a cross-sectional study', *BMC Family Practice*, 20: 1 (2019): https://pubmed.ncbi.nlm.nih.gov/31122187/

7   Souhail Alouini, Sejla Memic and Annabelle Couillandre, 'Pelvic floor muscle training for urinary incontinence with or without biofeedback or electrostimulation in women: a systematic review', *International Journal of Environmental Research and Public Health*, 19: 5 (2022): https://pubmed.ncbi.nlm.nih.gov/35270480/

8   Laura Geggel, 'Why Do You Pee When You're Nervous?', *Live Science* (2017): https://www.livescience.com/60524-why-do-you-pee-when-nervous.html

9   NHS England (2022), https://www.england.nhs.uk/2022/07/dame-deborah-james-helps-more-people-check-signs-of-cancer/

6: Supporting Your Breasts Well

1   Alexandra Milligan, Chris Mills, Jo Corbett et al., 'The influence of breast support on torso, pelvis and arm kinematics during a five kilometer treadmill run', *Human Movement Science*, 42 (2015), pp. 246–60: https://www.sciencedirect.com/science/article/abs/pii/S0167945715000925?via%3Dihub

2   J. White and J. Scurr, 'Evaluation of professional bra fitting criteria for bra selection and fitting in the UK', *Ergonomics*, 55: 6 (2012), pp. 704–11: https://www.tandfonline.com/doi/abs/10.1080/00140139.2011.647096?journalCode=terg2

3   Celeste Coltman, Julie R. Steele and Deirdre E. McGhee, 'Effect of aging on breast skin thickness and elasticity: implications for breast support', *Skin Research and Technology*, 23: 3 (2016), pp. 303–11: https://onlinelibrary.wiley.com/doi/10.1111/srt.12335

4   Joanna Scurr, Wendy Hedger, Paul Morris et al., 'The prevalence, severity, and impact of breast pain in the general population', *The Breast Journal*, 20: 5 (2014), pp. 508–13: https://onlinelibrary.wiley.com/doi/10.1111/tbj.12305

5   Brooke R. Brisbine, Julie R. Steele, Elissa J. Phillips et al., 'Breast and torso characteristics of female contact football players: implications for the design of sports bras and breast protection', *Ergonomics*, 63: 7 (2020), pp. 850–63: https://www.tandfonline.com/doi/full/10.1080/00140139.2020.1757161

6   Nicola Brown, Jennifer White, Amanda Brasher et al., 'The experience of breast pain (mastalgia) in female runners of the 2012 London Marathon and its effect on exercise behaviour', *British Journal of Sports Medicine*, 48: 4 (2014), pp. 320–25: https://bjsm.bmj.com/content/48/4/320

7   Deirdre E. McGhee and Julie R. Steele, 'Biomechanics of breast support for active women', *Exercise and Sport Sciences Reviews*, 48: 3 (2020), pp. 99–109: https://journals.lww.com/acsm-essr/fulltext/2020/07000/biomechanics_of_breast_support_for_active_women.1.aspx

8   Celeste E. Coltman, Julie R. Steele and Deirdre E. McGhee, 'Does breast size affect how women participate in physical activity?', *Journal of Science and Medicine in Sport*, 22: 3 (2019), pp. 324–9: https://www.jsams.org/article/S1440-2440(18)30875-2/fulltext

9   Ibid.

10   Timothy A. Exell, Alexandra Milligan, Jenny Burbage et al., 'There are two sides to every story: implications of asymmetry on breast support requirements for sports bra manufacturers', *Sports Biomechanics*, 20: 7 (2019), pp. 866–78: https://www.tandfonline.com/doi/abs/10.1080/14763141.2019.1614654?journalCode=rspb20

11   Kelly-Ann Page and Julie R. Steele, 'Breast motion and sports brassiere design', *Sports Medicine*, 27: 4 (1999), pp. 205–11: https://link.springer.com/article/10.2165/00007256-199927040-00001

12   Debbie Risius, Alexandra Milligan, Jason Berns et al., 'Understanding key performance indicators for breast support: an analysis of breast support effects on biomechanical, physiological and subjective measures during running', *Journal of Sports Sciences*, 35: 9 (2017), pp. 842–51: https://www.tandfonline.com/doi/abs/10.1080/02640414.2016.1194523?journalCode=rjsp20

13   Nathaniel A. Bates, Kevin R. Ford, Gregory D. Myer et al., 'Impact differences in ground reaction force and center of mass between the first and second landing phases of a drop vertical jump and their implications for injury risk assessment', *Journal of Biomechanics*, 46: 7 (2013), pp. 1237–41: https://www.sciencedirect.com/science/article/abs/pii/S0021929013001048?via%3Dihub

14   Alexandra Milligan, Chris Mills and Joanna Scurr, 'The effect of breast support on upper body muscle activity during 5 km treadmill running', *Human Movement Science*, 38 (2014), pp. 74–83: https://www.sciencedirect.com/science/article/abs/pii/S0167945714000906?via%3Dihub

15   J. White, H. Lunt, J. Scurr, 'The effect of breast support on ventilation and breast comfort perception at the onset of exercise', in Proceedings of the BASES annual conference. BASES, Essex (2011).

16   Alexandra Milligan et al., 'The influence of breast support on torso, pelvis and arm kinematics during a five kilometer treadmill run', op. cit.

17   Brooke R. Brisbine, Julie R. Steele, Elissa J. Phillips et al., 'The occurrence, causes and perceived performance effects of breast injuries in elite female athletes', *Journal of Sports Science & Medicine*, 18: 3 (2019), pp. 569–76: https://www.ncbi.nlm.nih.gov/pmc/articles/PMC6683617/

18   'Does Boob Protection Really Matter?', *Book Armour*, https://www.boobarmour.com.au/why-boob-armour/

19   Brooke R. Brisbine et al., 'Breast and torso characteristics of female
      contact football players', op. cit.

20   Examples of vests specifically designed for women who play contact
      sports available here: https://zenasport.co

7: Bodies that Move Well

1   Stephanie Stockwell, Mike Trott, Mark Tully et al., 'Changes in
     physical activity and sedentary behaviours from before to during the
     COVID-19 pandemic lockdown: a systematic review', *BMJ Open Sport
     & Exercise Medicine*, 7: 1 (2021): e000960

2   Kate Power, 'The COVID-19 pandemic has increased the care burden
     of women and families', *Sustainability: Science, Practice and Policy*, 16: 1
     (2020), pp. 67–73: https://www.tandfonline.com/doi/full/10.1080/
     15487733.2020.1776561

3   Dhruv R. Seshadri, Mitchell L. Thom, Ethan R. Harlow et al., 'Case
     report: return to sport following the COVID-19 lockdown and its
     impact on injury rates in the German soccer league', *Frontiers in Sports
     and Active Living*, 3: 604226 (2021): https://www.frontiersin.org/
     articles/10.3389/fspor.2021.604226/full

4   Benjamin P. Raysmith and Michael K. Drew, 'Performance success
     or failure is influenced by weeks lost to injury and illness in elite
     Australian track and field athletes: a 5-year prospective study', *Journal
     of Science and Medicine in Sport*, 19: 10 (2016), pp. 778–83: https://
     www.jsams.org/article/S1440-2440(15)00764-1/fulltext

5   Joanne L. Parsons, Stephanie E. Coen and Sheree Bekke, 'Anterior
     cruciate ligament injury: towards a gendered environmental approach',
     British Journal of Sports Medicine, 55: 17 (2021), pp. 984–90: https://
     bjsm.bmj.com/content/55/17/984

6   Fiona Tomas and Katie Whyatt, 'Exclusive: FA take groundbreaking
     action to halt ACL injury epidemic in women's
     football', *Telegraph*, 20 April 2020: https://www.telegraph.
     co.uk/womens-sport/2020/04/20/fa-take-
     groundbreaking-action-halt-acl-injury-epidemic-womens/

7   Joanne L. Parsons et al., 'Anterior cruciate ligament injury: towards a
     gendered environmental approach', op. cit.

8   R. M. Queen, 'Infographic: ACL injury and recovery', *Bone & Joint
     Research*, 6: 11 (2017), p. 621–2: https://online.boneandjoint.org.uk/
     doi/full/10.1302/2046-3758.611.BJR-2017-0330

9   Kamil E. Barbour, Charles G. Helmick, Michael Boring et al., 'Vital signs: prevalence of doctor-diagnosed arthritis and arthritis-attributable activity limitation – United States, 2013–2015', Morbidity and Mortality Weekly Report, 66: 9 (2017), pp. 264–253.

10   Kay M. Crossley, Brooke E. Patterson, Adam G. Culvenor et al., 'Making football safer for women: a systematic review and meta-analysis of injury prevention programmes in 11 773 female football (soccer) players', British Journal of Sports Medicine, 54 (2020): pp. 1089–98: https://bjsm.bmj.com/content/54/18/1089

11   Jennifer Moriatis Wolf, Lisa Cannada, Ann E. Van Heest et al., 'Male and female differences in musculoskeletal disease', Journal of the American Academy of Orthopaedic Surgeons, 23: 6 (2015), pp. 339–47: https://journals.lww.com/jaaos/Fulltext/2015/06000/Male_and_Female_Differences_in_Musculoskeletal.3.aspx

12   C. Y. Wild, J. R. Steele and B. J. Munro, 'Why do girls sustain more anterior cruciate ligament injuries than boys?: a review of the changes in estrogen and musculoskeletal structure and function during puberty', Sports Medicine, 42: 9 (2012), pp. 733–49.

13   Mohammad-Jafar Emami, Mohammad-Hossein Ghahramani, Farzad Abdinejad et al., 'Q-angle: an invaluable parameter for evaluation of anterior knee pain', Archives of Iranian Medicine, 10: 1 (2007), pp. 24–6: https://pubmed.ncbi.nlm.nih.gov/17198449/

14   Mimi Zumwalt, 'Musculoskeletal injury and the exercising female', in Jacky Forsyth and Claire-Marie Roberts, eds., The Exercising Female: Science and its Application (Routledge, 2019), pp. 142–59.

15   FIFA: FIFA 11+ Workbook, https://www.yrsa.ca/wp-content/uploads/2019/11/pdf/Fifa11/11plus_workbook_e.pdf

16   Laura J. Huston and Edward M. Wojtys, 'Neuromuscular performance characteristics in elite female athletes', American Journal of Sports Medicine, 24: 4 (1996), pp. 427–36: https://journals.sagepub.com/doi/10.1177/036354659602400405

17   Robert A. Malinzak, Scott M. Colby, Donald T. Kirkendall et al., 'A comparison of knee joint motion patterns between men and women in selected athletic tasks', Clinical Biomechanics, 16: 5 (2001), pp. 438–45: https://www.clinbiomech.com/article/S0268-0033(01)00019-5/fulltext

18   Simone Araujo, Daniel Cohen and Lawrence Hayes, 'Six weeks of core stability training improves landing kinetics among female

capoeira athletes: a pilot study', *Journal of Human Kinetics*, 45: 1 (2015), pp. 27–37: https://sciendo.com/article/10.1515/hukin-2015-0004

19 Nkechinyere Chidi-Ogbolu and Keith Baar, 'Effect of estrogen on musculoskeletal performance and injury risk', *Frontiers in Physiology*, 9: 1834 (2018): https://www.frontiersin.org/articles/10.3389/fphys.2018.01834/full

20 Gregory D. Myer, Kevin R. Ford, Mark V. Paterno et al., 'The effects of generalized joint laxity on risk of anterior cruciate ligament injury in young female athletes', *American Journal of Sports Medicine*, 36: 6 (2008), p. 1073–80: https://journals.sagepub.com/doi/10.1177/0363546507313572

21 Masataka Deie, Yukie Sakamaki, Yoshio Sumen et al., 'Anterior knee laxity in young women varies with their menstrual cycle', *International Orthopaedics*, 26: 3 (2002), pp. 154–6: https://link.springer.com/article/10.1007/s00264-001-0326-0

22 Bruno T. Saragiotto, Carla Di Pierro and Alexandre D. Lopes, 'Risk factors and injury prevention in elite athletes: a descriptive study of the opinions of physical therapists, doctors and trainers', *Brazilian Journal of Physical Therapy*, 18: 2 (2014), pp. 137–43: https://www.scielo.br/j/rbfis/a/PCRqktXqC79jkpwN4rJfX4q/?lang=en

23 T. Soligard, G. Myklebust, K. Steffen et al., 'Comprehensive warm-up programme to prevent injuries in young female footballers: cluster randomised controlled trial', *British Medical Journal*, 337:a2469 (2008).

24 Kay M. Crossley et al., 'Making football safer for women', op. cit.

25 '15-minute sports warm up exercises – Prevent injury Enhance Performance program', Saint Peter's Healthcare System video, 2014: https://www.youtube.com/watch?v=ZrT-3_q-dVU&feature=youtu.be

26 Kathrin Steffen, Roald Bahr and Grethe Myklebust, 'ACL prevention in female football', *Aspetar Sports Medicine Journal*, 2 (2013): https://www.aspetar.com/journal/upload/PDF/201312206292.pdf

27 'Game changers: 7 exercises to prevent ACL injuries', Safe Kids Worldwide video, 30 July 2013: https://www.youtube.com/watch?v=xWBSf4BfKRk; https://youtu.be/ZrT-3_q-dVU

28 Lou Atkins, Robert West and Susan Michie, *The Behaviour Change Wheel: A Guide to Designing Interventions* (Silverback, 2014).

29 Shaun Scholes, *Health Survey for England 2016: Physical Activity in Adults*, NHS Digital, 2017: http://healthsurvey.hscic.gov.uk/media/63730/HSE16-Adult-phy-act.pdf

30 Jenni Bourque, 'Almost ¾ of women have been made to feel uncomfortable in a public gym, survey suggests', *DNA Lean*, 31 July 2021: https://www.dna-lean.co.uk/a/blog/womens-gym-survey

31 Chloe Gray, 'Weight training: why is there still a gender gym gap?', *Stylist*: https://www.stylist.co.uk/fitness-health/weightlifting-gender-gym-gap-strength-training-men-vs-women/356580

32 Christine Ahmed, Wanda Wilton and Keenan Pituch, 'Relations of strength training to body image among a sample of female university students', *Journal of Strength and Conditioning Research*, 16: 4 (2002), pp. 645–8: https://pubmed.ncbi.nlm.nih.gov/12423199/

33 Brett R. Gordon, Cillian P. McDowell and Mats Hallgren, 'Association of efficacy of resistance exercise training with depressive symptoms', *JAMA Psychiatry*, 65: 6 (2018), pp. 566–76: https://jamanetwork.com/journals/jamapsychiatry/article-abstract/2680311?redirect=true

34 Matthew J. Delmonico, Matthew C. Kostek, Neil A. Doldo et al., 'Effects of moderate-velocity strength training on peak muscle power and movement velocity: do women respond differently than men?', *Journal of Applied Physiology*, 99: 5 (2005), pp. 1712–8: https://journals.physiology.org/doi/full/10.1152/japplphysiol.01204.2004

35 Paul Ansdell, Kevin Thomas, Glyn Howatson et al., 'Contraction intensity and sex differences in knee-extensor fatigability', *Journal of Electromyography and Kinesiology*, 37 (2017), pp. 68–74: https://www.sciencedirect.com/science/article/abs/pii/S1050641117302333?via%3Dihub

36 Sandra K. Hunter, 'Sex differences and mechanisms of task-specific muscle fatigue', *Exercise and Sport Sciences Review*, 37: 3 (2009), pp. 113–22: https://journals.lww.com/acsm-essr/Fulltext/2009/07000/Sex_Differences_and_Mechanisms_of_Task_Specific.3.aspx

37 P. Ansdell, Callum G. Brownstein, Jakob Škarabot et al., 'Menstrual cycle-associated modulations in neuromuscular function and fatigability of the knee extensors in eumenorrheic women', *Journal of Applied Physiology*, 126: 6 (2019), pp. 1701–12: https://journals.physiology.org/doi/full/10.1152/japplphysiol.01041.2018

38 Phillip Bishop, Kirk Cureton and Mitchell Collins, 'Sex difference in muscular strength in equally-trained men and women', *Ergonomics*, 30: 4 (1987), pp. 675–87: https://pubmed.ncbi.nlm.nih.gov/3608972/

39   Brandon M. Roberts, Greg Nuckols and James W. Krieger, 'Sex differences in resistance training: a systematic review and meta-analysis', *Journal of Strength and Conditioning Research*, 34: 5 (2020), pp. 1448–60. doi: https://journals.lww.com/nsca-jscr/Fulltext/2020/05000/Sex_Differences_in_Resistance_Training__A.30.aspx

40   Chang Woock Lee, Mark A. Newman and Steven E. Riechman, 'Oral contraceptive use impairs muscle gains in young women', *FASEB Journal*, 23: S1 (2009), pp. 955.25–955.25: https://faseb.onlinelibrary.wiley.com/doi/10.1096/fasebj.23.1_supplement.955.25

8: Eating Well

1   Lars T. Fadnes, Jan-Magnus Økland, Øystein A. Haaland et al., 'Estimating impact of food choices on life expectancy: a modeling study,' *PLOS Medicine*, 19: 3 (2022): https://journals.plos.org/plosmedicine/article?id=10.1371/journal.pmed.1003889

2   Sarah R. Davy, Beverly A. Benes and Judy A. Driskell, 'Sex differences in dieting trends, eating habits, and nutrition beliefs of a group of midwestern college students', *Journal of the Academy of Nutrition and Dietetics*, 106: 10 (2006), pp. 1673–7: https://www.jandonline.org/article/S0002-8223(06)01715-9/fulltext

3   Eva Wiseman, 'The truth about men, women and food', *Guardian*, 17 October 2010: https://www.theguardian.com/lifeandstyle/2010/oct/17/gender-eating-men-women

4   'Sports nutrition market worldwide from 2018 to 2025', *Statista*: https://www.statista.com/statistics/450168/global-sports-nutrition-market/#:~:text=The%20global%20sports%20nutrition%20market,billion%20U.S.%20dollars%20by%202023.&text=Sports%20nutrition%20products%20are%20designed,nutrients%20depleted%20during%20the%20workout

5   José L. Areta and Kirsty J. Elliott-Sale, 'Nutrition for female athletes: what we know, what we don't know, and why', *European Journal of Sport Science*, 22: 5 (2022), pp. 669–71: https://www.tandfonline.com/doi/full/10.1080/17461391.2022.2046176

6   Nathalie Boisseau and Laurie Isacco, 'Substrate metabolism during exercise: sexual dimorphism and women's specificities', *European Journal of Sports Science*, 22: 5 (2022), pp. 672–83: https://www.tandfonline.com/doi/abs/10.1080/17461391.2021.1943713?journalCode=tejs20

7 Edwina H. Yeung, Cuilin Zhang, Sunni L. Mumford et al., 'Longitudinal study of insulin resistance and sex hormones over the menstrual cycle: the BioCycle Study', *Journal of Clinical Endocrinology & Metabolism*, 95: 12 (2010), pp. 5435–42: https://academic.oup.com/jcem/article/95/12/5435/2835335?login=false

8 Stacy T. Sims, 'Sport-Specific Refueling' in *Roar: How to Match Your Food and Fitness to Your Unique Female Physiology for Optimum Performance, Great Health, and a Strong, Lean Body for Life* (Rodale, 2016).

9 Andrew R. Jagim, Jennifer Fields, Meghan K. Magee et al., 'Contributing factors to low energy availability in female athletes: a narrative review of energy availability, training demands, nutrition barriers, body image and disordered eating', *Nutrients*, 14: 5 (2022), p. 986: https://www.mdpi.com/2072-6643/14/5/986

10 Joan Eckerson, 'Energy and the nutritional needs of the exercising female', in Jacky Forsyth and Claire-Marie Roberts, eds., *The Exercising Female: Science and its Application* (Routledge, 2019), pp. 44–65.

11 Margo Mountjoy, Jorunn Kaiander Sundot-Borgen, Louise M. Burke et al., 'IOC consensus statement on relative energy deficiency in sport (RED-S): 2018 update', *British Journal of Sports Medicine*, 52: 11 (2018), pp. 687–97: https://bjsm.bmj.com/content/52/11/687

12 Joan Eckerson, 'Energy and the nutritional needs of the exercising female', op. cit.

13 John L. Ivy, 'Regulation of muscle glycogen repletion, muscle protein synthesis and repair following exercise', *Journal of Sports Science & Medicine*, 3: 3 (2004), pp. 131–8: https://www.ncbi.nlm.nih.gov/pmc/articles/PMC3905295/

14 I. L. Fahrenholtz, A. Sjödin, D. Benardot et al., 'Within-day energy deficiency and reproductive function in female endurance athletes', *Scandinavian Journal of Medicine and Science in Sports*, 28: 3 (2018), pp. 1139–46: https://onlinelibrary.wiley.com/doi/10.1111/sms.13030

15 Louise M. Burke, Gregory R. Cox, Nicola K. Cummings et al., 'Guidelines for daily carbohydrate intake: do athletes achieve them?', *Sports Medicine*, 31: 4 (2001), pp. 267–99: https://link.springer.com/article/10.2165/00007256-200131040-00003

16 James C. Morehen, Christopher Rosimus, Bryce P. Cavanagh et al., 'Energy expenditure of female international standard soccer players: a doubly labeled water investigation', *Medicine & Science in Sports & Exercise*, 54: 5 (2021), pp. 769–79:

https://journals.lww.com/acsm-msse/Abstract/2022/05000/
Energy_Expenditure_of_Female_International.7.aspx

17   Joan Eckerson, 'Energy and the nutritional needs of the exercising female', op. cit.

18   Mark Hargreaves, John A. Hawley and Asker Jeukendrup, 'Pre-exercise carbohydrate and fat ingestion: effects on metabolism and performance', *Journal of Sports Sciences*, 22: 1 (2004), pp. 31–8: https://doi.org/10.1080/0264041031000140536

19   M. A. Tarnopolsky, S. A. Atkinson, S. M. Phillips et al., 'Carbohydrate loading and metabolism during exercise in men and women', *Journal of Applied Physiology*, 78: 4 (1995), pp. 1360–8: https://journals.physiology.org/doi/abs/10.1152/jappl.1995.78.4.1360

20   M. A. Tarnopolsky, C. Zawada, L. B. Richmond et al., 'Gender differences in carbohydrate loading are related to energy intake', *Journal of Applied Physiology*, 91: 1 (2001), pp. 225–30: https://journals.physiology.org/doi/full/10.1152/jappl.2001.91.1.225

21   Joan Eckerson, 'Energy and the nutritional needs of the exercising female', op. cit.

22   Donald K. Layman, ' "Dietary Guidelines" should reflect new understandings about adult protein needs', *Nutrition and Metabolism*, 6: 12 (2009): https://nutritionandmetabolism.biomedcentral.com/articles/10.1186/1743-7075-6-12

23   Ralf Jäger, Chad M. Kerksick, Bill I. Campbell et al., 'International Society of Sports Nutrition position stand: protein and exercise', *Journal of the International Society of Sports Nutrition*, 14: 20 (2017): https://jissn.biomedcentral.com/articles/10.1186/s12970-017-0177-8

24   Kevin D. Tipton, Blake B. Rasmussen, Sharon L. Miller et al., 'Timing of amino acid–carbohydrate ingestion alters anabolic response of muscle to resistance exercise', *American Journal of Physiology: Endocrinology and Metabolism*, 281: 2 (2001), e197–206: https://journals.physiology.org/doi/full/10.1152/ajpendo.2001.281.2.E197

25   J. S. Volek, C. E. Forsythe and W. J. Kraemer, 'Nutritional aspects of women strength athletes', *British Journal of Sports Medicine*, 40: 9 (2006), pp. 742–8: https://bjsm.bmj.com/content/40/9/742

26   D. Enette Larson-Meyer, Bradley R. Newcomer and Gary R. Hunter, 'Influence of endurance running and recovery diet on intramyocellular lipid content in women: a ^{1}H NMR study', *American Journal of Physiology: Endocrinology and Metabolism*, 282: 1

(2002), e95–106: https://journals.physiology.org/doi/full/10.1152/ajpendo.2002.282.1.E95

27 Joan Eckerson, 'Energy and the nutritional needs of the exercising female', op. cit.

28 J. Décombaz, M. Fleith, H. Hoppeler et al., 'Effect of diet on the replenishment of intramyocellular lipids after exercise', *European Journal of Nutrition*, 39: 6 (2000), pp. 244–7: https://link.springer.com/article/10.1007/s003940070002

29 Heather Hendrick Fink and Alan E. Mikesky, *Practical Applications in Sports Nutrition*, 5th edn. (Jones and Bartlett, 2017).

30 D. Travis Thomas, Kelly Anne Erdman and Louise L. Burke, 'Position of the Academy of Nutrition and Dietetics, Dietitians of Canada, and the American College of Sports Medicine: nutrition and athletic performance', *Journal of the Academy of Nutrition and Dietetics*, 116: 3 (2016), pp. 501–28: https://www.jandonline.org/article/S2212-2672(15)01802-X/fulltext

31 K. A Wroble, M. N. Trott, G. G. Schweitzer et al., 'Low-carbohydrate, ketogenic diet impairs anaerobic exercise performance in exercise-trained women and men: a randomized-sequence crossover trial', *Journal of Sports Medicine and Physical Fitness*, 59: 4 (2019).

32 Stacy T. Sims, *Roar*, Chapter 10, pp. 166

33 Jessica do Nascimento Queiroz, Rodrigo Cauduro Oliveira Macedo, Grant M. Tinsley et al., 'Time-restricted eating and circadian rhythms: the biological clock is ticking', *Critical Reviews in Food Science and Nutrition*, 61: 17 (2021), pp. 2863–75: https://www.tandfonline.com/doi/abs/10.1080/10408398.2020.1789550?journalCode=bfsn20

34 Karen Van Proeyen, Karolina Szlufcik, Henri Nielens et al., 'Beneficial metabolic adaptations due to endurance exercise training in the fasted state', *Journal of Applied Physiology*, 110: 1 (2011), pp. 236–45. doi: https://journals.physiology.org/doi/full/10.1152/japplphysiol.00907.2010

35 Brad Schoenfeld, 'Does cardio after an overnight fast maximize fat loss?', *Strength and Conditioning Journal*, 33: 1 (2011), pp. 23–5: https://journals.lww.com/nsca-scj/fulltext/2011/02000/does_cardio_after_an_overnight_fast_maximize_fat.3.aspx

36 T. P. Aird, R. W. Davies and B. P. Carson, 'Effects of fasted vs fed-state exercise on performance and post-exercise metabolism: a systematic review and meta-analysis', *Scandinavian Journal of Medicine & Science*

in Sports, 28: 5 (2018), pp. 1476–93: https://onlinelibrary.wiley.com/doi/10.1111/sms.13054

37   Tasuku Terada, Saeed Reza Toghi Eshghi, Yilina Liubaoerjijin et al., 'Overnight fasting compromises exercise intensity and volume during sprint interval training but improves high-intensity aerobic endurance', *Journal of Sports Medicine and Physical Fitness*, 59: 3 (2018), pp. 357–65: https://pubmed.ncbi.nlm.nih.gov/29619796/

38   I. L. Fahrenholtz et al., 'Within-day energy deficiency and reproductive function in female endurance athletes', op. cit.

39   Kirsty J. Elliott-Sale, Adam S. Tenforde, Allyson L. Parziale et al., 'Endocrine effects of relative energy deficiency in sport', *International Journal of Sport Nutrition and Exercise*, 28: 4 (2018), pp. 335–49: https://journals.humankinetics.com/view/journals/ijsnem/28/4/article-p335.xml

40   Charles R. Pedlar, Carlo Brugnara, Georgie Bruinvels et al., 'Iron balance and iron supplementation for the female athlete: a practical approach', *European Journal of Sport Science*, 18: 2 (2018), pp. 295–305: https://www.tandfonline.com/doi/abs/10.1080/17461391.2017.1416178?journalCode=tejs20

41   Kelly A. Rossi, 'Nutritional aspects of the female athlete', *Clinics in Sports Medicine*, 36: 4 (2017), pp. 627–53: https://pubmed.ncbi.nlm.nih.gov/28886819/

42   Joan Eckerson, 'Energy and the nutritional needs of the exercising female', op. cit.

43   Emilly Martinelli Rossi, Renata Andrade Ávila, Maria Tereza W. D. Carneiro et al., 'Chronic iron overload restrains the benefits of aerobic exercise to the vasculature', *Biological Trace Element Research*, 198: 2 (2020), pp. 521–34: https://link.springer.com/article/10.1007/s12011-020-02078-y

44   D. Travis Thomas et al., 'Position of the Academy of Nutrition and Dietetics, Dietitians of Canada, and the American College of Sports Medicine: nutrition and athletic performance', op. cit.

45   Elizabeth Bertone-Johnson, Susan E. Hankinson, Adrianne Bendich et al., 'Calcium and vitamin D intake and risk of incident premenstrual syndrome', *Archives of Internal Medicine*, 165: 11 (2005), pp. 1246–52: https://jamanetwork.com/journals/jamainternalmedicine/fullarticle/486599

46   Guy B. Mulligan and Angelo Licata, 'Taking vitamin D with the largest meal improves absorption and results in higher serum levels

of 25-hydroxyvitamin D', *Journal of Bone and Mineral Research*, 25: 4 (2010), pp. 928–30: https://asbmr.onlinelibrary.wiley.com/doi/10.1002/jbmr.67

47   Kunling Wang, Hongyan Wei, Wanqi Zhang et al., 'Severely low serum magnesium is associated with increased risks of positive anti-thyroglobulin antibody and hypothyroidism: a cross-sectional study', *Science Reports*, 8: 1 (2018), p. 9904: https://www.nature.com/articles/s41598-018-28362-5

48   Stella Lucia Volpe, 'Magnesium and the athlete', *Current Sports Medicine Reports*, 14: 4 (2015), pp. 279–83: https://journals.lww.com/acsm-csmr/Fulltext/2015/07000/Magnesium_and_the_Athlete.8.aspx

49   Lara Briden, *Period Repair Manual: Natural Treatment for Better Hormones and Better Periods*, 1st edn. (Greenpeak Publishing, 2017).

50   Magdalena D. Cuciureanu and Robert Vink, 'Magnesium and stress', in Robert Vink and Mihai Nechifor, eds., *Magnesium in the Central Nervous System* (University of Adelaide Press, 2011): https://www.ncbi.nlm.nih.gov/books/NBK507250/

51   D. Travis Thomas et al., 'Position of the Academy of Nutrition and Dietetics, Dietitians of Canada, and the American College of Sports Medicine: nutrition and athletic performance', op. cit.

52   Batool Teimoori, Ghasemi Marzieh, Zeinab Sada Amir Hoseini et al., 'The efficacy of zinc administration in the treatment of primary dysmenorrhea', *Oman Medical Journal*, 31: 2 (2016), pp. 107–11: https://www.omjournal.org/articleDetails.aspx?coType=1&aId=743

53   Mark Jamieson, 'EIS help athletes manage illness over the holiday season', English Institute of Sport, 18 December 2018: https://eis2win.co.uk/article/eis-help-athletes-manage-illness-over-the-holiday-season/

54   Pooja Saigal and Damian Hanekom, 'Does zinc improve symptoms of viral upper respiratory tract infection?', *Evidence-Based Practice*, 23: 1 (2020), pp. 37–9: https://journals.lww.com/ebp/Citation/2020/01000/Does_zinc_improve_symptoms_of_viral_upper.32.aspx

55   Neil P. Walsh, 'Nutrition and athlete immune health: new perspectives on an old paradigm', *Sports Medicine*, 49: S2 (2019), pp. 153–68: https://link.springer.com/article/10.1007/s40279-019-01160-3

56   'Gut health & Covid-19: eating to support gut health and immunity', Zoe Health Study (2020): https://covid.joinzoe.com/post/gut-health-immunity-covid

57 Beibei Yang, Jinbao Wei, Peijun Ju et al., 'Effects of regulating intestinal microbiota on anxiety symptoms: a systematic review', *General Psychiatry*, 32: 2 (2019), p. e100056: https://gpsych.bmj.com/content/32/2/e100056

58 James M. Baker, Layla Al-Nakkash and Melissa M. Herbst-Kralovetz, 'Estrogen–gut microbiome axis: physiological and clinical implications', *Maturitas*, 103 (2017), pp. 45–53: https://www.maturitas.org/article/S0378-5122(17)30650-3/fulltext

59 Tanja Sobko, Suisha Liang, Will H. G. Cheng et al., 'Impact of outdoor nature-related activities on gut microbiota, fecal serotonin, and perceived stress in preschool children: the Play&Grow randomized controlled trial', *Scientific Reports*, 10: 21993 (2020): https://www.nature.com/articles/s41598-020-78642-2

60 Mike Amaranthus and Bruce Allyn, 'Healthy soil microbes, healthy people', *Atlantic*, 11 June 2013: https://www.theatlantic.com/health/archive/2013/06/healthy-soil-microbes-healthy-people/276710/

61 Patricia M. Barnes, Barbara Bloom, Richard L Nahin et al., 'Costs of complementary and alternative medicine (CAM) and frequency of visits to CAM practitioners, United States', *National Center for Health Statistics* (2009) National health statistics reports, 18: (PHS) 2009-1250: https://stacks.cdc.gov/view/cdc/11548

62 Peter Clarys, Tom Deliens, Inge Huybrechts et al., 'Comparison of nutritional quality of the vegan, vegetarian, semi-vegetarian, pesco-vegetarian and omnivorous diet', *Nutrients*, 6: 3 (2014), pp. 1318–32: https://www.mdpi.com/2072-6643/6/3/1318

63 'Relative energy deficiency in sport (RED-S)', Perth Sports Medicine: https://www.perthsportsmedicine.com.au/relative-energy-deficiency-in-sport-perth-claremont-cockburn-wa.html

64 Margot Mountjoy, Jorunn Sundgot-Borgen, Louise Burke et al., 'The IOC consensus statement: beyond the Female Athlete Triad – Relative Energy Deficiency in Sport (RED-S)', *British Journal of Sports Medicine*, 48: 7 (2014), pp. 491–7: https://bjsm.bmj.com/content/48/7/491?hootPostID=0116e43013bf35a19d2c4f30c76050b1

65 Dave C. Sona and Martin Fisher, 'Relative energy deficiency in sport (RED-S)', *Current Problems in Pediatric and Adolescent Health Care*, 52: 8 (2022)

66 Anne B. Loucks, Bentie Kiens and Hattie H. Wright, 'Energy availability in athletes', *Journal of Sports Science*, 29, supplement 1

(2011), pp. S7–15: https://www.tandfonline.com/doi/abs/10.1080/02640414.2011.588958?journalCode=rjsp20

9: Sleeping Well

1   N. P. Walsh, Shona L. Halson, Charli Sargent et al., 'Sleep and the athlete: narrative review and 2021 expert consensus recommendations', *British Journal of Sports Medicine*, 55 (2021), pp. 356–68: https://bjsm.bmj.com/content/55/7/356

2   Luke Gupta, Kevin Morgan and Sarah Gilchrist, 'Does elite sport degrade sleep quality? A systematic review', *Sports Medicine*, 47: 7 (2017), pp. 1317–33: https://link.springer.com/article/10.1007/s40279-016-0650-6

3   Helen S. Driver and Sheila R. Taylor, 'Exercise and sleep', *Sleep Medicine Reviews*, 4: 4 (2000), pp. 387–402: https://www.sciencedirect.com/science/article/abs/pii/S1087079200901102?via%3Dihub

4   John D. Chase, Paul A. Roberson, Michael J. Saunders et al., 'One night of sleep restriction following heavy exercise impairs 3-km cycling time-trial performance in the morning', *Applied Physiology, Nutrition, and Metabolism (Physiologie Appliquée, Nutrition et Métabolisme)*, 42: 9 (2017), pp. 909–15: https://cdnsciencepub.com/doi/10.1139/apnm-2016-0698

5   E. Van Caute, M. Kerkhofs, A. Caufriez et al., 'A quantitative estimation of growth hormone secretion in normal man: reproducibility and relation to sleep and time of day', *Journal of Clinical Endocrinology & Metabolism*, 74: 6 (1992), pp. 1441–50: https://academic.oup.com/jcem/article-abstract/74/6/1441/2655467?redirectedFrom=fulltext

6   Andrew M. Watson, 'Sleep and athletic performance', *Current Sports Medicine Reports*, 16: 6 (2017), pp. 413–18: https://journals.lww.com/acsm-csmr/fulltext/2017/11000/sleep_and_athletic_performance.11.aspx

7   Cheri D. Mah, Kenneth E. Mah, Eric J. Kezirian et al., 'The effects of sleep extension on the athletic performance of collegiate basketball players', *Sleep*, 34: 7 (2011), pp. 943–50: https://www.ncbi.nlm.nih.gov/pmc/articles/PMC3119836/

8   Hugh H. K. Fullagar, Sabrina Skorski, Rob Duffield et al., 'Sleep and athletic performance: the effects of sleep loss on exercise performance, and physiological and cognitive responses to exercise', *Sports Medicine*,

45: 2 (2015), pp. 161–86: https://link.springer.com/article/10.1007/
s40279-014-0260-0

9   Samuel J. Oliver, Ricardo J. S. Costa, Stewart J. Laing et al., 'One
      night of sleep deprivation decreases treadmill endurance performance',
      European Journal of Applied Physiology, 107: 2 (2009), pp. 155–61:
      https://link.springer.com/article/10.1007/s00421-009-1103-9

10   L. A. Reyner and J. A. Horne, 'Sleep restriction and serving accuracy
      in performance tennis players, and effects of caffeine', *Physiology &
      Behavior*, 120 (2013), pp. 93–6: https://www.sciencedirect.com/
      science/article/abs/pii/S0031938413002370?via%3Dihub

11   Jennifer Schwartz and Richard D. Simon Jr., 'Sleep extension improves
      serving accuracy: a study with college varsity tennis players', *Physiology
      & Behavior*, 151 (2015), pp. 541–4: https://www.sciencedirect.com/
      science/article/abs/pii/S0031938415300895?via%3Dihub

12   Matthew D. Milewski, David L. Skaggs, Gregory A. Bishop
      et al., 'Chronic lack of sleep is associated with increased
      sports injuries in adolescent athletes', *Journal of Pediatric
      Orthopaedics*, 34: 2 (2014), pp. 129–33: https://journals.
      lww.com/pedorthopaedics/Fulltext/2014/03000/
      Chronic_Lack_of_Sleep_is_Associated_With_Increased.1.aspx

13   P. von Rosen, A. Frohm, A. Kottorp et al., 'Multiple factors explain
      injury risk in adolescent elite athletes: applying a biopsychosocial
      perspective', *Scandinavian Journal of Medicine & Science in Sports*, 7:
      12 (2017), pp. 2059–60: https://onlinelibrary.wiley.com/doi/10.1111/
      sms.12855

14   Matthew Walker, *Why We Sleep: The New Science of Sleep and Dreams*
      (Penguin, 2018).

15   'Seven hours of sleep is optimal in middle and old age, say
      researchers', University of Cambridge, 28 April 2022:
      https://www.cam.ac.uk/research/news/seven-hours-
      of-sleep-is-optimal-in-middle-and-old-age-say-researchers

16   Gregory W. Kirschen, Jason J. Jones and Lauren Hale, 'The impact
      of sleep duration on performance among competitive athletes: a
      systematic literature review', *Clinical Journal of Sport Medicine*,
      30: 5 (2020), pp. 503–12: https://pubmed.ncbi.nlm.nih.gov/
      29944513/

17   Spencer Stuart Haines Roberts, Wei-Peng Teo and Stuart Anthony
      Warmington, 'Effects of training and competition on the sleep of
      elite athletes: a systematic review and meta-analysis', *British Journal*

of *Sports Medicine*, 53: 8 (2019), pp. 513–22: https://bjsm.bmj.com/content/53/8/513

18   Ibid.

19   Kelley Pettee Gabriel, Barbara Sternfeld, Eric J. Shiroma et al., 'Bidirectional associations of accelerometer-determined sedentary behavior and physical activity with reported time in bed: women's health study', *Sleep Health*, 3: 1 (2017), pp. 49–55: https://www.sciencedirect.com/science/article/abs/pii/S2352721816300882?via%3Dihub

20   Petros G. Botonis, Nickos Koutouvakis and Argyris G. Toubekis, 'The impact of daytime napping on athletic performance – a narrative review', *Scandinavian Journal of Medicine & Science in Sports*, 31: 12 (2021), pp. 2164–77: https://onlinelibrary.wiley.com/doi/10.1111/sms.14060

21   Elisabeth Petit, Fabienne Mougin, Hubert Bourdin et al., 'A 20-min nap in athletes changes subsequent sleep architecture but does not alter physical performances after normal sleep or 5-h phase-advance conditions', *European Journal of Applied Physiology*, 114 (2014), pp. 305–15: https://link.springer.com/article/10.1007/s00421-013-2776-7

22   Tom Deboer, 'Sleep homeostasis and the circadian clock: do the circadian pacemaker and the sleep homeostat influence each other's functioning?', *Neurobiology of Sleep and Circadian Rhythms*, 5 (2018), pp. 68–77: https://www.sciencedirect.com/science/article/pii/S2451994417300068?via%3Dihub

23   Shannon O'Donnell, Christopher M. Beaven and Matthew Driller, 'The influence of match-day napping in elite female netball athletes', *International Journal of Sports Physiology and Performance*, 13: 9 (2018), pp. 1143–8: https://journals.humankinetics.com/view/journals/ijspp/13/9/article-p1143.xml

24   Hugh H. K. Fullagar et al., 'Sleep and athletic performance: the effects of sleep loss on exercise performance, and physiological and cognitive responses to exercise', op. cit.

25   Daniel A. Cohen, Wei Wang, James K. Wyatt et al., 'Uncovering residual effects of chronic sleep loss on human performance', *Science Translational Medicine*, 2: 14 (2010), pp. 14ra3: https://www.science.org/doi/10.1126/scitranslmed.3000458

26   A.T. Mulgrew, G. Nasvadi, A. Butt et al., 'Risk and severity of motor vehicle crashes in patients with obstructive sleep apnoea/hypopnoea', *Thorax*, 63: 6 (2008), pp. 536–41

27   'Driving drowsy vs. driving drunk: the fatal mistake most people make', *Advanced Sleep Medicine Services Inc*: https://www.sleepdr.com/the-sleep-blog/driving-drowsy-vs-driving-drunk-the-fatal-mistake-most-people-make/

28   F.P. Cappuccio, L. D'Elia, P. Strazzullo et al., 'Sleep duration and all-cause mortality: a systematic review and meta-analysis of prospective studies', *Sleep*, 33: 5 (2010), pp. 585–92. doi: 10.1093/sleep/33.5.585.

29   Jennifer Soong, 'How sleep loss affects women more than men', *WebMD*, 15 February 2010: https://www.webmd.com/sleep-disorders/features/how-sleep-loss-affects-women-more-than-men

30   Danielle Pacheco, 'Do women need more sleep than men?', *Sleep Foundation*, 6 May 2022: https://www.sleepfoundation.org/women-sleep/do-women-need-more-sleep-than-men

31   Monica P. Mallampalli and Christine L. Carter, 'Exploring sex and gender differences in sleep health: a Society for Women's Health Research Report', *Journal of Women's Health*, 23: 7 (2014), pp. 553–62: https://www.liebertpub.com/doi/10.1089/jwh.2014.4816

32   David A. Kalmbach, Thomas Roth, Phillip Cheng et al., 'Mindfulness and nocturnal rumination are independently associated with symptoms of insomnia and depression during pregnancy', *Sleep Health*, 6: 2 (2020), pp. 185–91: https://www.sciencedirect.com/science/article/pii/S2352721819302621?via%3Dihub

33   Zawn Villines, 'How to stop ruminating thoughts', *Medical News Today*, 8 November 2019: https://www.medicalnewstoday.com/articles/326944#tips

34   Franziska C. Weber, Heidi Danker-Hopfe, Ezgi Dogan-Sander et al., 'Restless legs syndrome prevalence and clinical correlates among psychiatric inpatients: a multicenter study', *Frontiers in Psychiatry*, 13, 846165 (2022): https://www.frontiersin.org/articles/10.3389/fpsyt.2022.846165/full

35   'Restless legs syndrome: causes', NHS: https://www.nhs.uk/conditions/restless-legs-syndrome/causes/

36   Martino F. Pengo, Christine H. Won and Ghada Bourjeily, 'Sleep in women across the life span', *Chest*, 154: 1 (2018), pp. 196–206: https://journal.chestnet.org/retrieve/pii/S0012369218305701

37   Alanna Dorsey, Luis de Lecea and Kimberly J. Jennings, 'Neurobiological and hormonal mechanisms regulating women's sleep',

Frontiers in Neuroscience, 14: 625397 (2021): https://www.frontiersin. org/articles/10.3389/fnins.2020.625397/full#B162

38   S. Nowakowski, J. Meers and E. Heimbach, 'Sleep and Women's Health', *Sleep Medicine Research*, 4: 1 (2013), pp. 1–22.

39   Martino F. Pengo et al., 'Sleep in women across the life span', op. cit.

40   John C. Stevenson, Arkadi Chines, Kaijie Pan et al., 'A pooled analysis of the effects of conjugated estrogens/bazedoxifene on lipid parameters in postmenopausal women from the Selective Estrogens, Menopause, and Response to Therapy (SMART) Trials', *Journal of Clinical Endocrinology and Metabolism*, 100: 6 (2015), pp. 2329–38: https:// academic.oup.com/jcem/article/100/6/2329/2829631?login=false

41   'Are you struggling to sleep?', Greenway Community Practice: https:// www.greenwaycommunitypractice.nhs.uk/insomnia

42   Ashley Richmond, 'Why we should wake up at the same time every day', *Medium*, 26 January 2017: https:// medium.com/in-fitness-and-in-health/why-we- should-wake-up-at-the-same-time-every-day-889a4815447a

43   Katherine Gillen, '25 healthy midnight snacks for late night munching, according to a nutritionist', *PureWow*, 4 December 2021: https:// www.purewow.com/food/healthy-midnight-snacks

44   Bahar Gholipour, 'Sleeping pills: older adults more likely to use', *Live Science*, 29 August 2013: https://www.livescience.com/39278- americans-use-prescription-sleeping-pills.html

45   Neil Breen and Jonathan Marshall, 'Swimming legend Grant Hackett admits he used sleeping pill Stillnox for longer than usual period', *Fox Sports*, 28 September 2022: https://www.foxsports. com.au/more-sports/swimming-legend-grant-hackett-admits- he-used-sleeping-pill-stillnox-for-longer-than-usual-period/ news-story/79d93590f2a73f35b4446079669c75a7

46   'Australia's Olympic athletes banned from taking sleeping medication from time of selection, says AOC', *ABC News*, 28 August 2015: https://www.abc.net.au/news/2015-08-28/ aussies-athletes-banned-from-sleeping-pills/6733600

47   'How to access insomnia treatment on the NHS', *Sleepstation* (2022), https://www.sleepstation.org.uk/articles/sleep-clinic/ nhs-options-for-insomnia-treatments/

48   Allison T. Siebern and Rachel Manber, 'New developments in cognitive behavioral therapy as the first-line treatment of insomnia',

Psychology Research and Behavior Management, 4 (2011), pp. 21–8: https://www.ncbi.nlm.nih.gov/pmc/articles/PMC3218784/

49   Jamie Millar, 'Five scientifically proven ways to improve your sleep', *Mr Porter* (2022), https://www.mrporter.com/en-gb/journal/lifestyle/five-expert-tips-improve-better-sleep-routine-exercise-10388884

50   Eric Suni, 'Sleep diary', *Sleep Foundation*, 12 April 2022: https://www.sleepfoundation.org/sleep-diary

51   Karen Zraick and Sarah Mervosh, 'The sleep tracker that could make your insomnia worse', *New York Times*, 13 June 2019: https://www.nytimes.com/2019/06/13/health/sleep-tracker-insomnia-orthosomnia.html

10: A Woman's Brain

1   Leanne Norman and Jamie French, 'Understanding how high performance women athletes experience the coach–athlete relationship', *International Journal of Coaching Science*, 7: 1 (2013), pp. 3–24: https://www.semanticscholar.org/paper/Understanding-how-High-Performance-Women-Athletes-Norman-French/12ad213a4973efae47b72e4324401a4ade95cbf5

2   Sarah McKay, *Demystifying the Female Brain: A Neuroscientist Explores Health, Hormones and Happiness* (Orion Spring, 2018).

3   Tara Swart, *The Source: Open Your Mind, Change Your Life* (Vermillion, 2020).

4   Stephanie A. Shields, *Speaking from the Heart: Gender and the Social Meaning of Emotion* (Cambridge University Press, 2002).

5   Kateri McRae, Kevin N. Ochsner, Iris B. Mauss et al., 'Gender differences in emotion regulation: an fMRI study of cognitive reappraisal', *Group Processes & Intergroup Relations*, 11: 2 (2008), pp. 143–62: https://journals.sagepub.com/doi/10.1177/1368430207088035

6   David Nield, 'Women's brains have more blood flow than men's, new study shows', *Science Alert*, 8 August 2017: https://www.sciencealert.com/women-s-brains-are-more-active-than-men-s-shows-a-new-study

7   Simon Baron-Cohen, 'The empathising-systemising theory of autism: implications for education', *Tizard Learning Disability Review*, 14: 3 (2009), pp. 4–13: https://www.researchgate.net/publication/

239781577_The_empathising-systemising_theory_of_autism_
Implications_for_education

8   Amber D. Mosewich, Adrianne B. Vangool, Kent C. Kowalski et al.,
     'Exploring women track and field athletes' meanings of muscularity',
     Journal of Applied Sport Psychology, 21: 1 (2009), pp. 99–115:
     https://www.tandfonline.com/doi/abs/10.1080/
     10413200802575742

9   Félix Guillén and Rosaura Sánchez, 'Competitive anxiety in expert
     female athletes: sources and intensity of anxiety in National Team
     and First Division Spanish basketball players', *Perceptual and Motor
     Skills*, 109: 2 (2009), pp. 407–19: https://journals.sagepub.com/
     doi/10.2466/pms.109.2.407-419

10   S. D. Hoar, K. C. Kowalski, P. Gaudreau et al., *A Review of Coping in
     Sport* (2006), Literature Reviews in Sport Psychology (pp. 47–90),
     New York: Nova Science Publishers.

11   Megan M. Kelly, Audrey R. Tyrka, Lawrence H. Price et al., 'Sex
     differences in the use of coping strategies: predictors of anxiety and
     depressive symptoms', *Depression and Anxiety*, 25: 10 (2008), pp. 839–
     46: https://onlinelibrary.wiley.com/doi/10.1002/da.20341

12   'N. Ireland coach apologises for saying women's players "more
     emotional" than men', *Reuters*, 13 April 2022: https://www.reuters.
     com/lifestyle/sports/n-ireland-coach-slammed-saying-womens-
     players-more-emotional-than-men-2022-04-13/

13   'How to keep your head in the game: sports psychology tips & more',
     Sports Illustrated video, 2 October 2017: https://www.youtube.com/
     watch?v=4clEOMwTTcM

14   'Box breathing relaxation technique: how to calm feelings of stress or
     anxiety' video, Sunnybrook Hospital, 5 October 2020: https://www.
     youtube.com/watch?v=tEmt1Znux58

15   Ami Strutin Belinoff, 'Mental resetting in competition',
     Bridge Blog, 15 April 2017: https://blog.bridgeathletic.com/
     mental-resetting-in-competition

16   Dana R. Carney, Amy J. C. Cuddy and Andy J. Yap, 'Power posing:
     brief nonverbal displays affect neuroendocrine levels and risk tolerance',
     Psychological Science, 21: 10 (2010), pp. 1363–8.

17   Shelley E. Taylor, 'Tend and befriend: biobehavioral bases of affiliation
     under stress', *Current Directions in Psychological Science*, 15: 6 (2006),
     pp. 273–7: https://journals.sagepub.com/doi/10.1111/j.1467-
     8721.2006.00451.x

18 Anjula Razdan, 'Are women more likely to "tend and befriend"?', *Experience Life*, 1 November 2007: https://experiencelife.com/article/tend-and-befriend/

19 'Loneliness and social isolation linked to serious health conditions', Centers for Disease Control and Prevention: https://www.cdc.gov/aging/publications/features/lonely-older-adults.html

20 Katty Kay and Claire Shipman, 'The confidence gap', *Atlantic*, May 2014: https://www.theatlantic.com/magazine/archive/2014/05/the-confidence-gap/359815/

21 Meghan Huntoon, Amanda Durik and Maura Dooley, 'Women and self-promotion: a test of three theories', *Psychological Reports*, 122: 1 (2019), pp. 219–30: https://www.researchgate.net/publication/322766624_Women_and_Self-Promotion_A_Test_of_Three_Theories

22 Hanna Hart, 'The confidence gap is a myth, but double standard does exist: how women can navigate', *Forbes*, 5 March 2019: https://www.forbes.com/sites/hannahart/2019/03/05/the-confidence-gap-is-a-myth-but-a-double-standard-does-exist-how-women-can-navigate/

23 Claire-Marie Roberts, Leah Ferguson and Amber Mosewich, 'The psychology of female sport performance', in Jacky Forsyth and Claire-Marie Roberts, eds., *The Exercising Female: Science and its Application* (Routledge, 2019), pp. 175–86.

24 Kate Hays, Owen Thomas, Ian Maynard et al., 'The role of confidence in world-class sport performance', *Journal of Sports Sciences*, 27: 11 (2009), pp. 1185–99.

25 Kate Hays, Ian Maynard, Owen Thomas et al., 'Sources and types of confidence identified by world class sport performers', *Journal of Applied Sport Psychology*, 19: 4 (2007), pp. 434–56: https://www.tandfonline.com/doi/abs/10.1080/10413200701599173

26 Leanne Norman and Jamie French, 'Understanding how high performance women athletes experience the coach–athlete relationship', op. cit.

27 Brené Brown, *The Gifts of Imperfection: Let Go of Who You Think You're Supposed to Be and Embrace Who You Are* (Hazelden, 2018).

28 Megan L. Olson and Paul Kwon, 'Brooding perfectionism: refining the roles of rumination and perfectionism in the etiology of depression', *Cognitive Therapy and Research*, 32 (2008), pp. 788–802: https://link.springer.com/article/10.1007/s10608-007-9173-7#article-info

29 Thomas Curran and Andrew P. Hill, 'Perfectionism is increasing over time: a meta-analysis of birth cohort differences from 1989 to 2016',

Psychological Bulletin, 145: 4 (2019), pp. 410–29: https://www.apa.org/pubs/journals/releases/bul-bul0000138.pdf

30   Brené Brown, *The Power of Vulnerability: Teachings on Authenticity, Connection and Courage* audiobook (Sounds True, 2013).

31   Daniel F. Gucciardi, Sheldon Hanton and Scott Fleming, 'Are mental toughness and mental health contradictory concepts in elite sport? A narrative review of theory and evidence', *Journal of Science and Medicine in Sport*, 20: 3 (2017), pp. 307–11: https://www.jsams.org/article/S1440-2440(16)30149-9/fulltext

32   Karin Hägglund, Göran Kenttä, Richard Thelwell et al., 'Is there an upside of vulnerability in sport? A mindfulness approach applied in the pursuit of psychological strength', *Journal of Sport Psychology in Action*, 10: 4 (2019), pp. 220–6: https://doi.org/10.1080/21520704.2018.1549642

33   Ibid.

34   Kristin Neff, 'Self-compassion: an alternative conceptualization of a healthy attitude toward oneself', *Self and Identity*, 2: 2 (2003), pp. 85–101: https://doi.org/10.1080/15298860309032

35   Ibid.

36   Amber Mosewich, 'Self-compassion in sport and exercise', in Gershon Tenenbaum and Robert C. Eklund, eds., *Handbook of Sports Psychology*, 4th edn. (Wiley, 2020): https://self-compassion.org/wp-content/uploads/2021/11/Mosewich-2020-Self-Compassion-in-Sport-and-Exercise.pdf

37   Amber D. Mosewich, Peter R. E. Crocker, Kent C. Kowalski et al., 'Applying self-compassion in sport: an intervention with women athletes', *Journal of Sport & Exercise Psychology*, 35: 5 (2013), pp. 514–24: https://delongis-psych.sites.olt.ubc.ca/files/2017/12/Applying-self-compassion-in-sport.pdf

38   Ibid.

39   Neil K. McGroarty, Symone M. Brown and Mary K. Mulcahey, 'Sport-related concussion in female athletes: a systematic review', *Orthopaedic Journal of Sports Medicine*, 8: 7 (2020), 2325967120932306: https://www.ncbi.nlm.nih.gov/pmc/articles/PMC7366411/

40   Paul McCrory, Willem Meeuwisse, Jiří Dvorak et al., 'Consensus statement on concussion in sport – the 5th international conference on concussion in sport held in Berlin, October 2016', *British Journal of Sports Medicine*, 51 (2018), pp. 838–47: https://bjsm.bmj.com/content/51/11/838

41   David Robson, 'Men and women aren't equal when it comes to concussion', *University of Colorado Anschutz Medical Campus*, 6 December 2019: https://medschool.cuanschutz.edu/center-for-womens-health-research/insights/news-articles/women's-health-articles/men-and-women-aren't-equal-when-it-comes-to-concussion

42   https://committees.parliament.uk/work/977/concussion-in-sport/news/156748/sport-allowed-to-mark-its-own-homework-on-reducing-concussion-risks/

43   The driving force behind Chronic Traumatic Encephalopathy (CTE), *Concussion Legacy Foundation*, https://concussionfoundation.org/cte-resources/subconcussive-impacts

44   Dr Emer MacSweeney, 'CTE: The silent killer in contact sports', *TEDx Athens* (2022): https://youtu.be/QXn-okL2rfs

45   K. A. Hagan, K. L. Munger, A. Ascherio et al., 'Epidemiology of major neurodegenerative diseases in women: contribution of the nurses' health study', *American Journal of Public Health*, 106: 9 (2016), pp. 1650–5.

46   Ryan T. Tierney, Michael R. Sitler, C. Buz Swanik et al., 'Gender differences in head–neck segment dynamic stabilization during head acceleration', *Medicine & Science in Sports & Exercise*, 37: 2 (2005), pp. 272–79: https://journals.lww.com/acsm-msse/Fulltext/2005/02000/Gender_Differences_in_Head_Neck_Segment_Dynamic.15.aspx

47   Kathryn Wunderle, Kathleen M. Hoeger, Erin Wasserman et al., 'Menstrual phase as predictor of outcome after mild traumatic brain injury in women', *Journal of Head Trauma Rehabilitation*, 29: 5 (2014), pp. e1–8: https://journals.lww.com/headtraumarehab/Fulltext/2014/09000/Menstrual_Phase_as_Predictor_of_Outcome_After_Mild.11.aspx

48   Ibid.

49   Jess Hayden, 'Long-term brain damage likely a significantly bigger issue in women's rugby than men's, says lead concussion doctor', *RugbyPass* (2020): https://www.rugbypass.com/news/long-term-brain-damage-could-be-a-significantly-bigger-issue-in-womens-rugby-than-mens-says-lead-concussion-doctor/

50   A headband designed to reduce concussive and sub-concussive brain injury. The first CE marked protective of its type across the UK and Europe. https://www.rezonwear.com/

51 T. Matsuura, Y. Takata, T. Iwame et al., 'Limiting the Pitch Count in Youth Baseball Pitchers Decreases Elbow Pain', *Orthopaedic Journal of Sports Medicine*, 9: 3 (2021)

11: Well Women, Across Our Lives

1   RCOG, *Better for Women Report* (2019): https://www.rcog.org.uk/better-for-women

2   Steve Biddulph, *10 Things Girls Need Most – To Grow Up Strong and Free* (Harper Thorsons, 2017).

3   Reframing Sport for Teenage Girls, Women in Sport (2019): https://womeninsport.org/research-and-advice/our-publications/reframing-sport-for-teenage-girls-building-strong-foundations-for-their-futures/

4   Atefeh Omrani, Joanna Wakefield-Scurr, Jenny Smith et al., 'Breast education improves adolescent girls' breast knowledge, attitudes to breasts and engagement with positive breast habits', *Frontiers in Public Health*, 8 (2020), 591927: https://www.frontiersin.org/articles/10.3389/fpubh.2020.591927/full

5   Royal College of Obstetricians and Gynaecologists, *Better for Women Report* (2019): https://www.rcog.org.uk/better-for-women

6   Sarah McKay, *Demystifying The Female Brain: A Neuroscientist Explores Health, Hormones and Happiness* (Orion Spring, 2018).

7   Sport England, 'Active Lives Children and Young People Survey, Academic Year 2018/19, Sport England', December 2019: https://sportengland-production-files.s3.eu-west-2.amazonaws.com/s3fs-public/2020-01/active-lives-children-survey-academic-year-18-19.pdf?VersionId=cVMsdnpBoqROViY6iiUjpQY6WcRyhtGs

8   Narelle Eather, Adrienne Bull, Myles D. Young et al., 'Fundamental movement skills: where do girls fall short? A novel investigation of object-control skill execution in primary-school aged girls', *Preventive Medicine Reports*, 11 (2018), pp. 191–5: https://www.sciencedirect.com/science/article/pii/S2211335518301025?via%3Dihub

9   L. L. Hardy, S. Mihrshahi, B. A. Drayton et al., 'NSW Schools Physical Activity and Nutrition Survey (SPANS) 2015: Full Report', NSW Department of Health, 2016.

10 Janet Shibley Hyde, 'The gender similarities hypothesis', *American Psychologist*, 60: 6 (2005), pp. 581–92: https://www.apa.org/pubs/journals/releases/amp-606581.pdf

11   'Females "less physically active"', *BBC News*, 6 January 2009: http://news.bbc.co.uk/1/hi/health/7811398.stm

12   'Changing the Game, for Girls', Women's Sport and Fitness Foundation: https://www.womeninsport.org/wp-content/uploads/2015/04/Changing-the-Game-for-Girls-Teachers-Toolkit.pdf

13   Peter C. Scales, Peter L. Benson and Eugene C. Roehlkepartain, 'Adolescent thriving: the role of sparks, relationships, and empowerment', *Journal of Youth and Adolescence*, 40: 3 (2011), pp. 263–77: https://link.springer.com/article/10.1007/s10964-010-9578-6

14   Steve Biddulph, *10 Things Girls Need Most*, op. cit.

15   'Landmark study: menopausal women let down by employers and healthcare providers', *Fawcett Society*, 2 May 2022: https://www.fawcettsociety.org.uk/news/landmark-study-menopausal-women-let-down-by-employers-and-healthcare-providers

16   Joyce C. Harper, Samantha Phillips, Vikram Talaulikar et al., 'An online survey of perimenopausal women to determine their attitudes and knowledge of the menopause', 2022: https://journals.sagepub.com/doi/10.1177/17455057221106890

17   'Perimenopause', *WebMD*: https://www.webmd.com/menopause/guide/guide-perimenopause

18   Grace Huang, Shehzad Basaria, Thomas Travison et al., 'Testosterone dose-response relationships in hysterectomized women with or without oophorectomy: effects on sexual function, body composition, muscle performance and physical function in a randomized trial', *Menopause*, 21: 6 (2014), pp. 612–23: https://journals.lww.com/menopausejournal/Abstract/2014/06000/Testosterone_dose_response_relationships_in.13.aspx

19   Shazia Jehan, Giardin Jean-Louis, Ferdinand Zizi et al., 'Sleep, melatonin, and the menopausal transition: what are the links?', *Sleep Science*, 10: 1 (2017), pp. 11–18: http://sleepscience.org.br/details/400

20   Mingyu Yi, Sixue Wang, Ting Wu et al., 'Effects of exogenous melatonin on sleep quality and menopausal symptoms in menopausal women: a systematic review and meta-analysis of randomized controlled trials', *Menopause*, 28: 6 (2021), pp. 717–25: https://journals.lww.com/menopausejournal/Abstract/2021/06000/Effects_of_exogenous_melatonin_on_sleep_quality.17.aspx

21 Elena Volpi, Reza Nazemi and Satoshi Fujita, 'Muscle tissue changes with aging', *Current Opinion in Clinical Nutrition and Metabolic Care*, 7: 4 (2004), pp. 405–10: https://doi.org/10.1097%2F01.mco.0000134362.76653.b2

22 Rosanne Woods, Rebecca Hess, Carol Biddington et al., 'Association of lean body mass to menopausal symptoms: the study of women's health across the nation', *Women's Midlife Health*, 6: 10 (2020): https://womensmidlifehealthjournal.biomedcentral.com/articles/10.1186/s40695-020-00058-9

23 Lori B. Forner, Emma M. Beckman and Michelle D. Smith, 'Symptoms of pelvic organ prolapse in women who lift heavy weights for exercise: a cross-sectional survey', *International Urogynecology Journal*, 31: 8 (2020), pp. 1551–58: https://pubmed.ncbi.nlm.nih.gov/31813038/

24 Linda Wasmer Andrews, 'How strength training helps keep anxiety at bay', *Psychology Today*, 29 March 2017: https://www.psychologytoday.com/gb/blog/minding-the-body/201703/how-strength-training-helps-keep-anxiety-bay

12: Where We Belong

1 'The Murphy's law of menstruation', *Free the Tampons*: https://www.freethetampons.org/uploads/4/6/0/3/46036337/ftt_infographic.pdf

2 Emily Peck, 'Free tampons should be a human right', *Free the Tampons*, 3 March 2016: https://www.freethetampons.org/free-tampons-should-be-a-human-right.html#

3 Claire Diamond, 'Period poverty: Scotland first in world to make period products free', *BBC News*, 15 August 2022: https://www.bbc.co.uk/news/uk-scotland-scotland-politics-51629880

4 We like the ones sold by FabLittleBag, at www.fablittlebag.com

5 'The Female Cricket Store: changing the landscape of women's cricket', the *Cricketer*, 17 June 2020: https://www.thecricketer.com/Topics/news/the_female_cricket_store_changing_the_landscape_of_womens_cricket.html

6 www.thefemalecricketstore.com

7 Anne Miltenburg, 'Kit that fits: developing women's sportswear', *Works That Work*: https://worksthatwork.com/9/kit-that-fits-developing-womens-sportswear

8   Hannah Norrish, Fiona Farringdon, Max Bulsara et al., 'The effect of school uniform on incidental physical activity among 10-year-old children', *Asia-Pacific Journal of Health, Sport and Physical Education*, 3: 1 (2012), pp. 51–63: https://www.tandfonline.com/doi/abs/10.1080/18377122.2012.666198

9   Jonathan Shaw, 'The deadliest sin', *Harvard Magazine*, March–April 2004: https://www.harvardmagazine.com/2004/03/the-power-of-exercise

10   Jazmin Sawyers, 'This is important. Period.', *Spikes*, 25 January 2018: https://spikes.worldathletics.org/post/jazmin-sawyers-talks-periods

11   Davina McCall, *Sex Myths and the Menopause*, Channel 4 (2021): https://www.channel4.com/programmes/davina-mccall-sex-myths-and-the-menopause

12   Brené Brown, 'The most dangerous stories we make up', *Brené Brown*, 27 July 2015: https://brenebrown.com/articles/2015/07/27/the-most-dangerous-stories-we-make-up/

Recommended Reading

Anstiss, Sue, *Game On, The Unstoppable Rise of Women's Sport*, Unbound, 2021

Atkins, Lou; West, Robert; Michie, Susan, *The Behaviour Change Wheel: A Guide to Designing Interventions*, Silverback, 2014

Biddulph, Steve, *10 Things Girls Need Most – To Grow Up Strong and Free*, Harper Thorsons, 2017

Briden, Lara, *Hormone Repair Manual: Every Woman's Guide to Healthy Hormones*, CreateSpace Independent Publishing Platform, 2017

Briden, Lara, *Period Repair Manual: Natural Treatment for Better Hormones and Better Periods*, Greenpeak Publishing, 2017

Brown, Brené, *The Gifts of Imperfection: Let Go of Who You Think You're Supposed to Be and Embrace Who You Are*, Hazelden, 2018

Brown, Brené, *The Power of Vulnerability: Teachings on Authenticity, Connection and Courage* audiobook, Sounds True, 2013

Clear, James, *Atomic Habits*, Random House Business, 2018

Criado Perez, Caroline, *Invisible Women: Exposing Data Bias in a World Designed for Men*, Chatto & Windus, 2013

Hill, Maisie, *Period Power*, Green Tree, 2019

Hill, Sarah, *How the Pill Changes Everything: Your Brain on Birth Control*, Orion Spring, 2019

Jackson, Gabrielle, *Pain and Prejudice; A Call to Arms for Women and Their Bodies*, Piatkus, 2019

McCall, Davina and Potter, Dr Naomi, *Menopausing, The Positive Roadmap to Your Second Spring*, HQ, 2022

McKay, Sarah, *Demystifying the Female Brain: A Neuroscientist Explores Health, Hormones and Happiness*, Orion Spring, 2018

Sims, Stacy T., *Roar: How to Match Your Food and Fitness to Your Unique Female Physiology for Optimum Performance, Great Health, and a Strong, Lean Body for Life*, Rodale, 2016

Shields, Stephanie A., *Speaking from the Heart: Gender and the Social Meaning of Emotion*, Cambridge University Press, 2002

Swart, Tara, *The Source: Open Your Mind, Change Your Life*, Vermillion, 2020

Switzer, Kathrine, *Marathon Woman*, Carroll & Graf, 2007

Walker, Matthew, *Why We Sleep: The New Science of Sleep and Dreams*, Penguin, 2018

Index

bigger breasts 122–4, 135
breast pain 54, 60, 121–2, 133, 271, 303
during puberty 261
effect of progesterone on 45
injuries 132, 133–5
movement of during activities 120, 121, 122, 124, 126, 130, 131–2
smaller breasts 124
teenage 124, 259, 261
see also bras
breathing: and breast movement 132
box breathing 233, 237
breathing exercises 222, 233, 237
breathlessness 59
mental resetting 233, 237
pelvic floor exercises 103–4, 105
Briden, Lara 191–2
bridge 152
British Menopause Society 277
Brown, Brené 242, 245

caffeine 70, 71, 194, 222, 225, 282
calcium 20, 190–1, 198, 199
calories, menstrual cycle and 44
Cambridge University 212
Canadian Running 98
carbohydrates 173–9, 180, 200
carb-loading 177–9
as exercise fuel 171, 177–9, 183, 187
how often and when to eat 174–7
ketogenic diets 185
limiting 169
and midlife 284
post-exercise 67–8, 171
which to eat 175–6
cardiovascular health 45, 88, 191, 203
carotenoids 197
cat naps 214–15
central nervous system 44, 144
cervical fluid 31
Charlton, Bobby 254
children: movement skills 268–9
weight training and 165
Chronic Traumatic Encephalopathy (CTE) 252–3, 255
Clear, James 8
clock lunge 151
clumsiness 70, 71

cognitive behavioural therapy for insomnia (CBT-I) 224
cognitive function 45, 88
the coil *see* intrauterine system (IUS)
collagen 68–9
COM-B model 154–6
communication gap 9
compassion 306
concussion, sports-related 10, 251–6
Concussion in Sport Group 251
conditioning 144, 153–4, 283
COM-B model 154–6
multi-component conditioning programmes 148–9
confidence 20, 240–2, 244, 248, 304, 306
constipation 57, 59, 112–14, 116
contraception 14–15, 54, 73–96
how to crack 96
myths 83–6
side effects 87–95
see also individual types of contraception
cooling down 138
Cooper's ligaments 119–20
coordination 69–70
the core 101, 144–5
corpus luteum 30–1
cortisol 89–90, 186, 188, 234, 238
courage 43, 306
Covassin, Professor Tracey 251–2
Covid-19 48, 136
cramps 191, 192
cricket 298
Cuddy, Amy 234
cycling 164, 211, 296–7

dairy 53
data gap 9–12
dead fat necrosis 133
dehydration 182, 183
dementia 252, 253, 254, 278
depression: perfectionism and 242
as side effect of the pill 92, 93
as sign of RED-S 201, 202
sleep and 217, 226
strength training and 158, 284
stress and 88
diaphragm 101, 106